THE
FOODCOMA
COOKBOOK

THE FOODCOMA COOKBOOK

JESSE FREEMAN

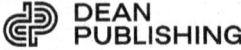

First published in 2023 by Dean Publishing
Copyright © Jesse Freeman
The moral right of the author has been asserted.

Editing and Creative Direction: Dean Publishing

ISBN: 978-1-925452-76-1

Category: COOKING/Methods/Barbecue & Grilling
COOKING/Special Ingredients/Burgers

This book is not intended as a substitute for nutritional, health, fitness or medical advice. The reader should regularly consult a physician or trained dietician in matters relating to their nutritional needs or general health. The ideas and recipes within this book are only the opinion of the author and are not intended to replace any medical or dietary advice or diagnose health issues or nutritional imbalances or needs.

This cookbook is based on the author's own nutritional preferences and experiences and not intended to persuade or influence the consumer in any way regarding matters of eating, health, nutrition or dietary recommendations. Food choices are unique and up to the individual. For professional advice, it is recommended to consult your physician.

The views and opinions expressed in this book are those of the author and do not necessarily reflect the official policy or position of any other agency, publisher, organization, employer or company. Assumptions made in the analysis are not reflective of the position of any entity other than the author(s)—and, these views are always subject to change, revision, and rethinking at any time. The author, publisher or organizations are not to be held responsible for misuse, reuse, recycled and cited and/or uncited copies of content within this book by others.

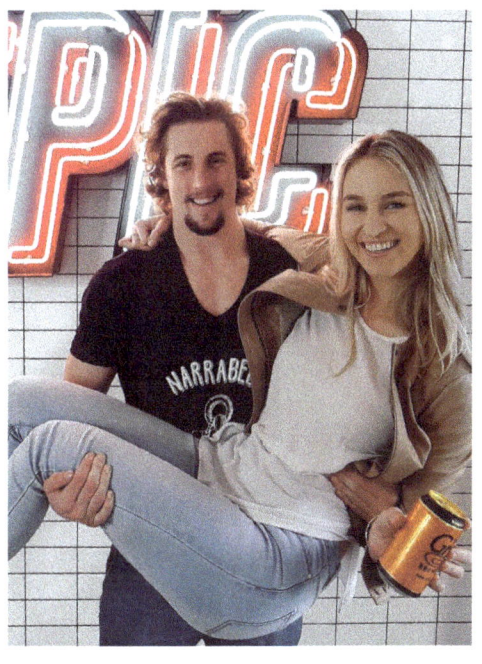

To my wonderful wife, Kira. These past couple years have been such a rollercoaster, and I appreciate and love your ongoing support and steadfast approach to my strange career. I hope my love for you can be immortalized in this book, along with the beautiful memories that brought us together.

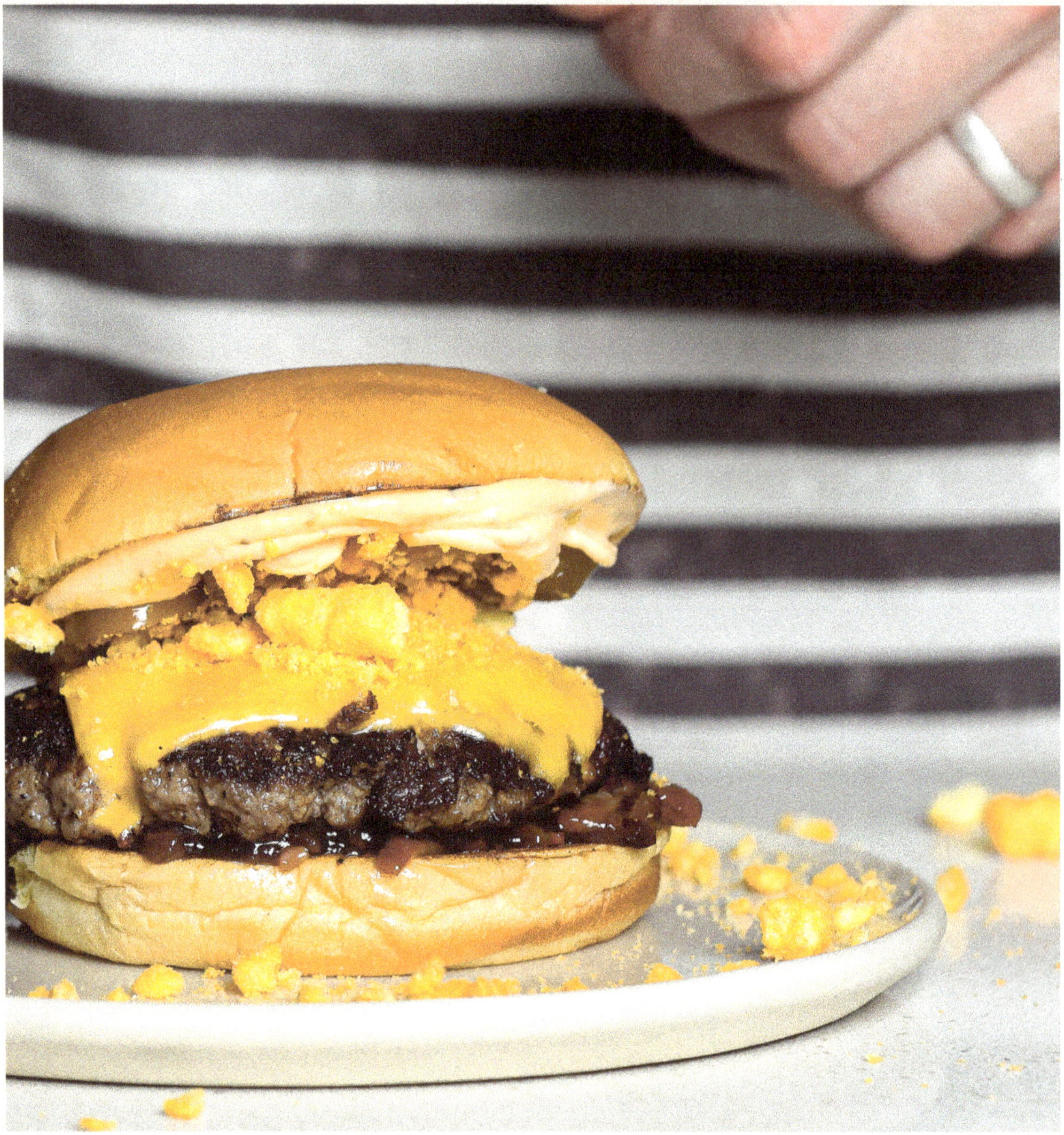

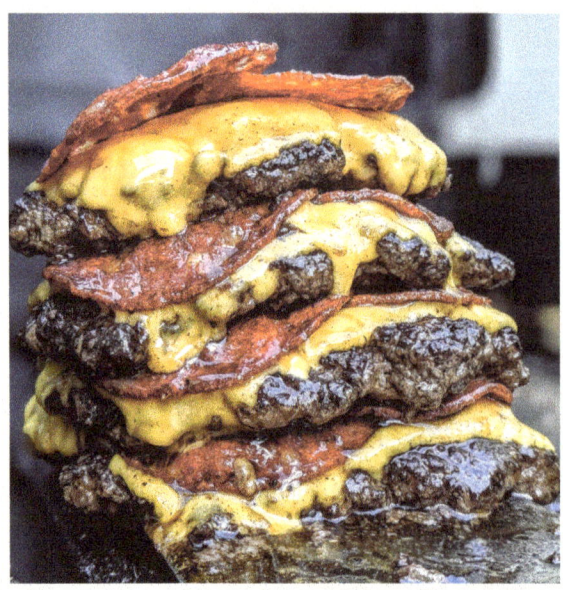
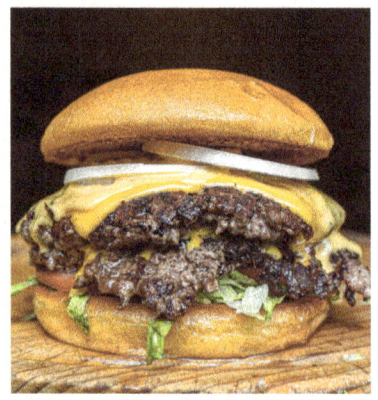

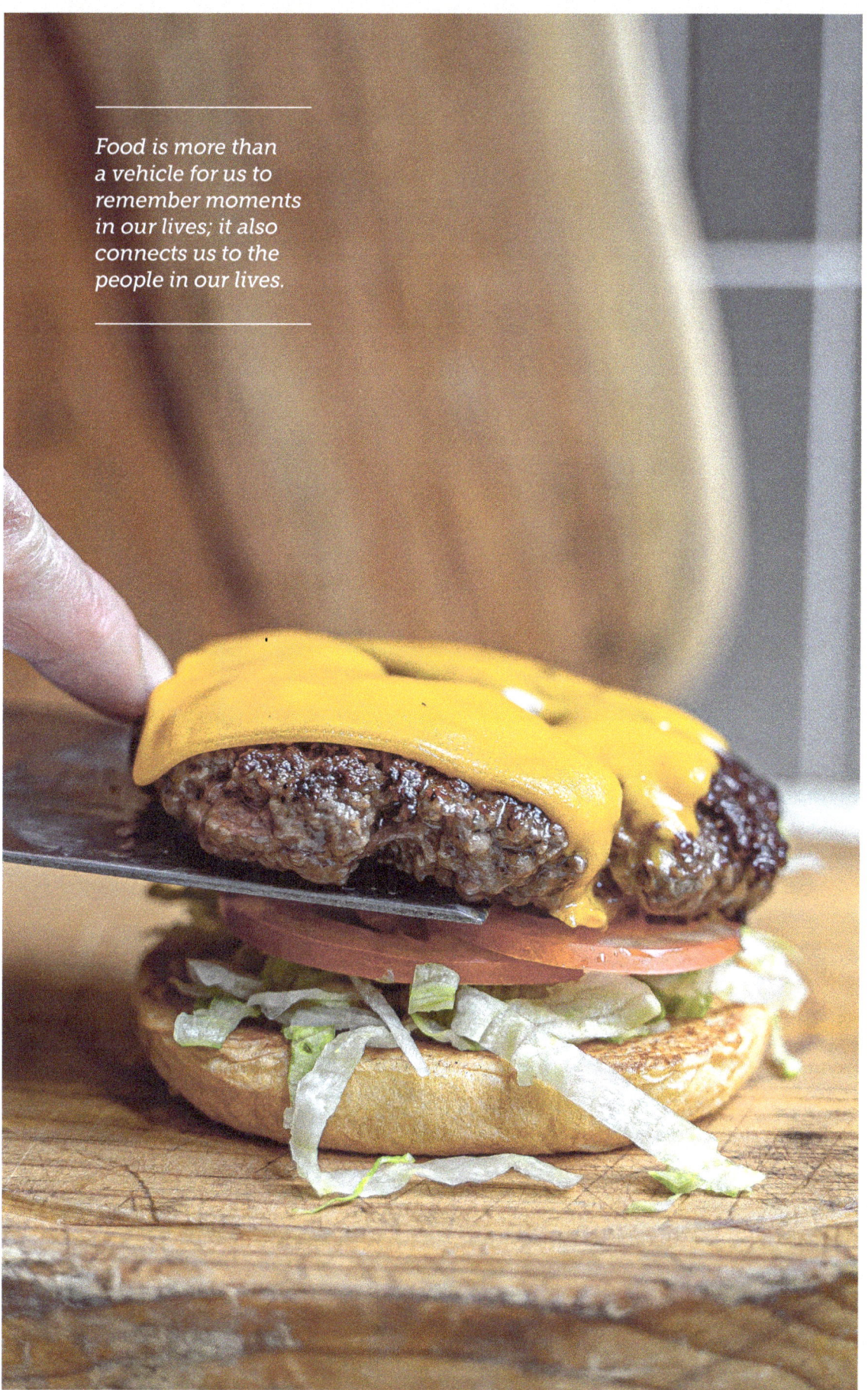

Food is more than a vehicle for us to remember moments in our lives; it also connects us to the people in our lives.

CONTENTS

INTRODUCTION..................................11

THE TOOLS 21

THE MEAT 29

THE SUPPORTING PLAYERS 37

THE SMASHING SYMPHONY 43

THE JOURNEY BEGINS..........................47

THE OG 48

THE OKLAHOMA STYLE SMASH....................52

THE HOMER SIMPSON 56

THE MEATLOVERS PIZZA 60

THE FAT FRYDAY..................................68

THE HOLY GUACAMOLE............................72

THE BACON ME CRAZY 76

THE OKTOBERFEST 80

THE SIMPLE SANDO...............................84

THE LANDCRUISER 90

THE STEAK SANDO................................94

THE GODFATHER...................................... 100

THE JUICY LUCY 104

THE 4:20 O'CLOCK..................................... 108

THE TRIPLE BYPASS.................................112

THE MONSTER MASH 116

THE MI-SO HUNGRY 120

THE HUM DINGER BUM STINGER.................124

THE DOWN UNDAAAAH 128

THE FINAL CHAPTER............................**132**
SPECIAL MENTIONS **134**
ACKNOWLEDGMENTS **154**
ABOUT THE AUTHOR **157**

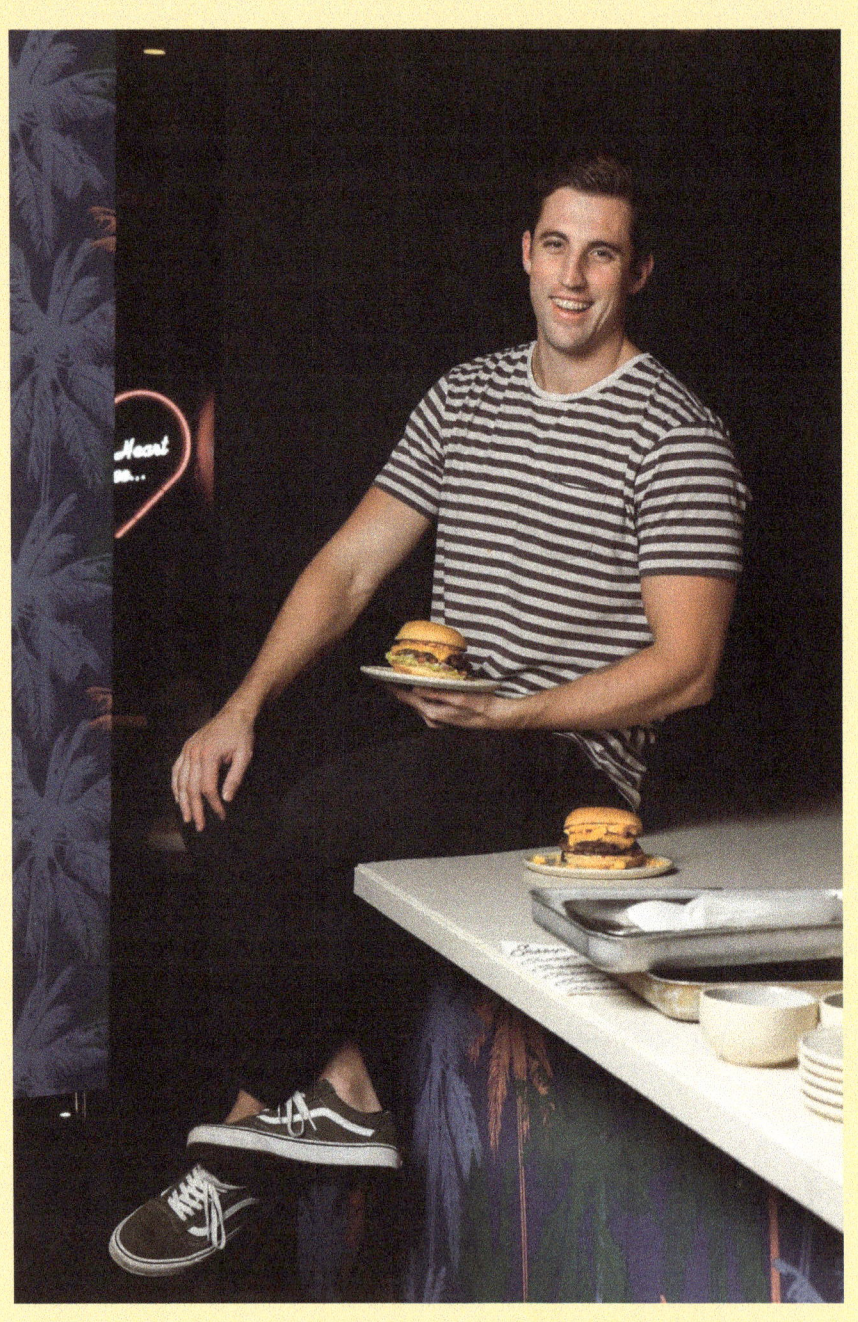

INTRODUCTION

It's so difficult to summarize something that has been a dominating figure throughout all of my journey. Sitting down and writing these words is such a labor of love; I find myself getting sentimental and nostalgic the deeper my thoughts travel through the topic of food. It's nearly impossible to define how monumental it has been in my life, but I'm going to give it my best shot.

I find it utterly beautiful that I can connect a food memory to almost every big moment in my life. It's such a powerful tool that helps timestamp the proverbial "feed" of your journey.

Food is deeply embedded in my first ever memories. As a young four-year-old boy, I remember traveling around Australia with my family, soaking up the culture, seeing the rawness of our country, and experiencing food. Every small glimpse is shaded with a memory of what I was eating at that moment. When we were swimming in an underground rock pool, I remember making a small shelter on the sand while eating mint slice. Camping underneath the starlit sky in the middle of the beach, I can still smell the freshness of a recently baked campfire damper. I can still remember sharing an ice-cold sprite with my older brother, Jamie, on a sweltering hot day in the Australian red desert.

> *Food has played such a pivotal and defining role in my life.*

Then life fast forwards. Suddenly, I'm learning French with some of my best childhood friends. Our amazing tutor, Jean Luc, brought such joy to our lives because we didn't just learn the language, but we had to do so while cooking French patisserie. We'd laugh and speak remnants of French, while deliciously sweet treats were being baked, and a distinct sweet aroma filled the air.

Within a blink of an eye, I'm in high school. I've picked up the sport of triathlon, marking a huge stage of my life. I'm waking up at 4:30 a.m., spending a nearly conversationless drive to my swimming squad with my dad (because we were both so tired), munching down on muesli bars trying to fuel myself up. I would spend Saturday mornings cycling, unknowingly building a relationship with a lifelong friend, Damo. We'd then hurry back to my parents' place and grill a whole kilogram of bacon, along with eight scrambled eggs. We'd blend up chocolate milkshakes and eat breakfast until we were sluggishly rolling out of the dining area. We'd also spend Friday night—after going for a "run," which ended up being us just kicking a footy around—punishing our hidden stash of V energy drinks, spoonfuls of dry Milo, and playing Battlefield on my PlayStation till late at night. But we don't speak about that to our parents.

We'd travel down to our triathlon coach—and incredible mentor—Mick, in Caringbah. Here we'd be tasked with cooking our own meals all weekend, as well as cooking for our coach. Safe to say there were some good meals (like our chicken nachos) and some terrible ones (that time we didn't know how to mash a potato). We'd also mark off the end of a hard race by driving the hour and a half back home together and stopping off for our mandatory KFC feast. Later in school, I took a year off racing to concentrate on studying. Instead of post-training meals, I'd sneak off during free periods—which were supposed to be study periods—with my other lifelong mates, Lochie and Liam, to smash a bag of gravy-covered chips at the local supermarket.

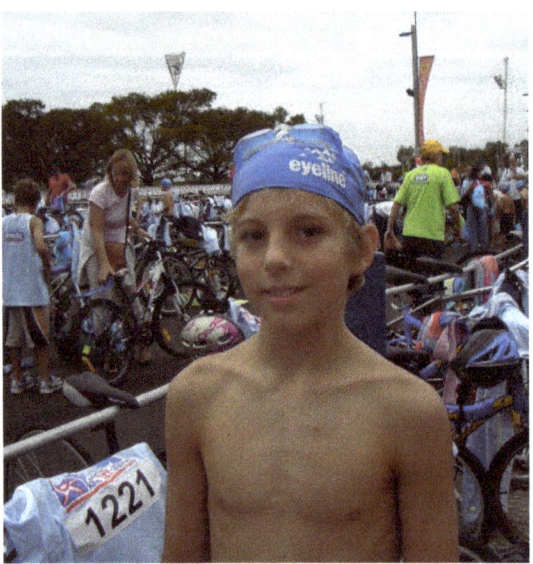
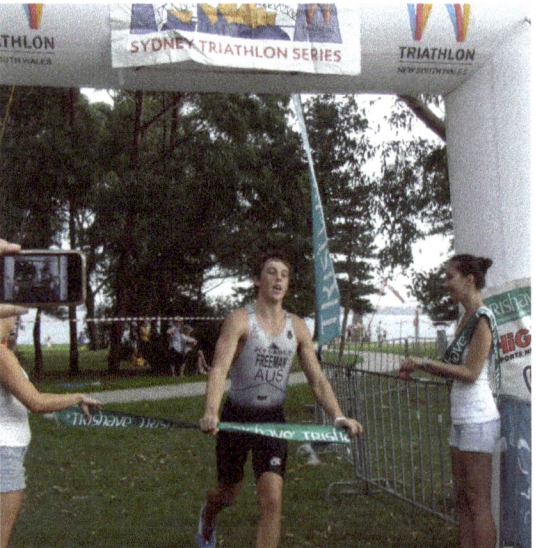

FINDING FOOD IN ALL THE RIGHT PLACES

Graduation was all a blur, and, soon after, I decided to move out of home. Wasting no time, I moved in with a couple of twenty-two year olds, Ben and Grant. Paying rent at eighteen years old, I couldn't afford my Saturday 1 kg of bacon. I wasn't exactly living like a king, but I look back on that time with nostalgia. I was working four jobs with minimal pay, but one job had a sweet sweet perk. As a Chinese food delivery driver, I would fang my old 1987 Mitsubishi Magna around the streets of the Northern Beaches, pumping tunes and wrestling with my lack of power steering. I'd be able to have my pick of a meal at the end of a shift. Without fail, my order was always a "large fried rice with satay chicken." I'd bring it home after a long, twelve-hour day of barely eating a thing and demolish it without saying a word to either of my roommates.

During the day, I'd work at Rebel Sport, slinging shoes to unsuspecting locals. I'd get a ten-minute break around 11 a.m., at which time I'd sprint down to the nearby Subway at breakneck speed, order my pizza sub with chipotle southwest sauce, and wolf it down within a couple of minutes. My pay would usually land on Tuesdays, and sometimes funds got real tight. So, Mondays could be a bit of a free-for-all. Usually, my lunch and dinner would consist of a $1 loaf of white bread and $3 Colby cheese, hopefully in grilled form if I had access to a grill.

Paying rent at eighteen years old, I couldn't afford my Saturday 1 kg of bacon.

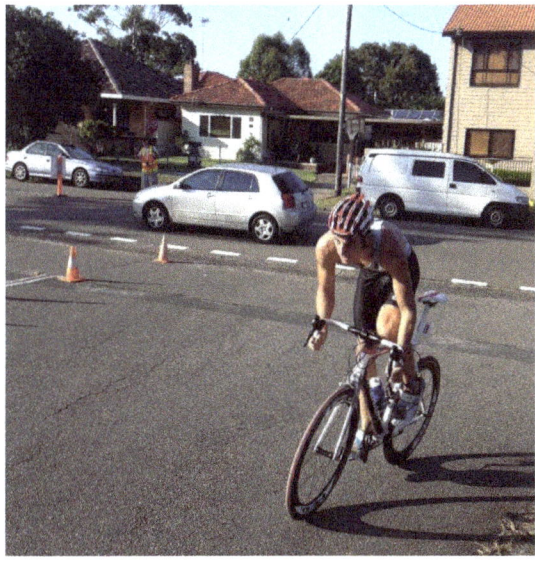

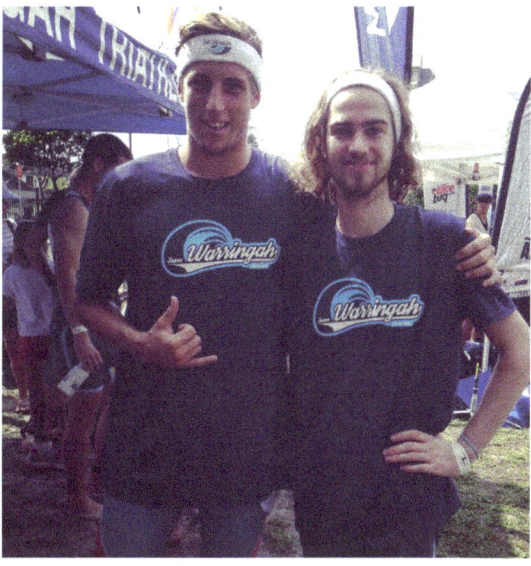

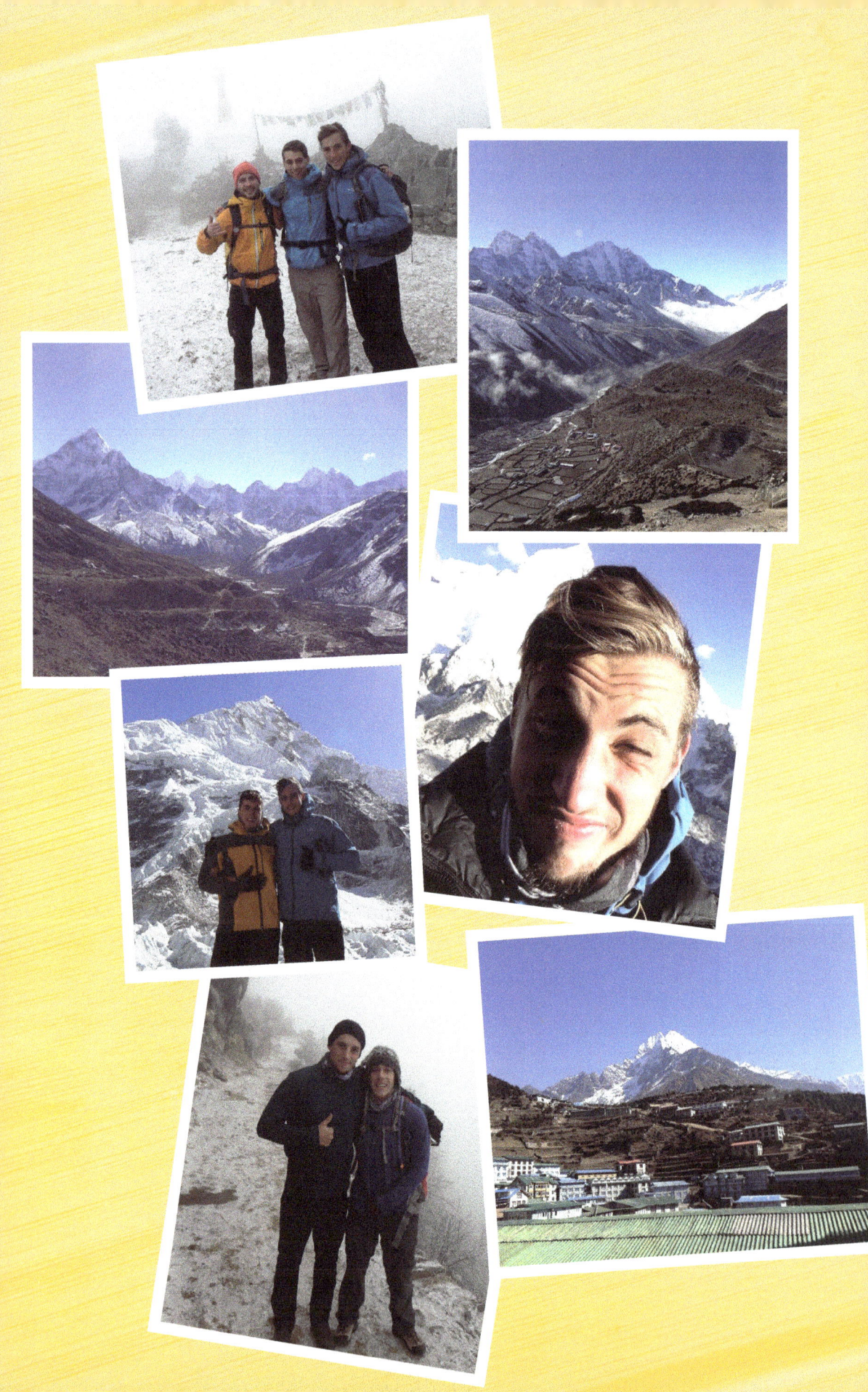

A TASTE OF THE WORLD

After a stint living out of home, I shamelessly moved back in with my parents to save for an overseas trip with Liam. Nepal and Thailand. We landed in Nepal, and our trip to the hotel felt like a delirious dream. After trying my luck with a squat toilet, which is an experience of its own, we grabbed our bags and attempted to hail a lift. The airport was rife with activity, locals shouting and trying to get our attention, people offering to take our bags, and us not being able to find our shuttle. We learned very quickly that everything had a price, so we tipped our way to the hotel and finally had our first meal.

We were the only people in our hotel's restaurant—if you could call it that—but our first meal felt like it was cooked by Gordan Ramsay himself. A simple chow mein and chicken curry, paired with a local Everest beer. Every mouthful was comfort and gave us the energy to drag ourselves upstairs. We both looked at each other and laughed, realizing we were drunk after a couple beers due to the altitude. We met our hiking group, and then it was all systems go on our journey up the mountain. We were very quickly introduced to dal bhat, which was dangerous for someone of my appetite. It was a vegetarian curry with a lentil soup, and the deal was simple. If you finished your plate, you could have a free refill, but you could not share with others. I took it as a challenge, with most of our stops ending with me three to four plates deep.

I'll never forget the beer we had on the highest day of our climb. We had decided to try and complete Everest Base Camp and Kala Patthar on the same day to avoid a 3 a.m. start the next morning. Everything went smooth for Everest Base Camp; my best mate and I achieved what we had set out to do. Elated from our victory, with energy still in the tank, we convinced the guide to let us do Kala Patthar. We started our climb up, and the air was so still. There was such a lack of life that we could hear our own heartbeats, and it felt like we were on another planet. Three of us made it to the top: me, an Englishman training for the army, and a local Sherpa.

We celebrated and took photos of the sunset, but the situation quickly started to turn sour. A strong wind swept through, knocking us left and right, alarmingly close to the edge of the mountain. We all grabbed one another and held ourselves tight, both for warmth and for stability. It seemed like it would never end; I hadn't experienced such violent winds in my entire life. Finally, it subsided, and we all looked at each other in shock … until I burst out laughing. We started to smile again and made our merry way down the mountain, only to find what we had left behind during our ascent. A few of the others had followed us. Some were okay, but a couple were absolutely shell-shocked to their core. We had to convince them to get off the ground, and we put our arms around them as we played Jack Johnson on a speaker to calm them down. What a journey. We finally made it to the bottom, the village of Gorakshep. We threw down our bags and congregated around the fire. I was offered a beer, and in my exhausted state, I couldn't say no. I started to drink it and within minutes, I was asleep, beaten by the mountain.

WHEN EATING GETS COMPETITIVE

I returned to Australia with a refreshed view on life. I started my university degree in commerce and after a couple years, I retired from triathlons and used my free time to surf every morning with another of my lifelong friends, Simo. I had already been surfing with him for years, but now it turned into a daily obsession. Hopping our way down the beaches, searching for the best waves, we'd shiver our way into our wet-from-the-day-before wetsuits until they were fully zipped up. We'd spend a couple of hours telling jokes, checking up on each other's mental health, and bonding on our outlooks on life. After jumping out of the water, cold to our cores, we'd find the nearest Bakers Delight and scoff down a couple of blueberry and white chocolate scones, paired with a choccy milk. We'd give each other a supportive slap on the ass and move on to our days, knowing that life couldn't get much better.

I'd consume over 2 kg of meat and veggies and go walking with my roommate.

Then came the chapter of competitive eating. This is the part of the story where you guys probably got introduced to me. After spending a few years chopping and changing my diet and exercise—that attention to detail triathlon itch needed to be scratched—and staying up late at night to read articles about nutrition, I eventually landed on intermittent fasting. It suited my lifestyle, and it gave me the flexibility to feast on food, rather than snack. Perfect. During the days of Pokémon Go, I'd consume over 2 kg of meat and veggies and go walking with my roommate, trying to find that damned Pikachu that seemed to be dodging us in our house. Eventually, after a long Saturday night, Lochie would dare me to eat a whole KFC Family Burger Box the next day. Always up for a challenge, I accepted, demolished it, and decided it wasn't enough—so I ate a frozen pizza as well. The next part of my life was a huge food-fueled blur.

Lochie gave me the push to start doing competitive eating. We traveled around Sydney—and once Melbourne—videoing me taking on some of the weirdest and biggest challenges. These became a small hit on YouTube, which then gave me the motivation to create an Instagram and document my everyday meals, as well as the challenges. This is when burgers became my obsession.

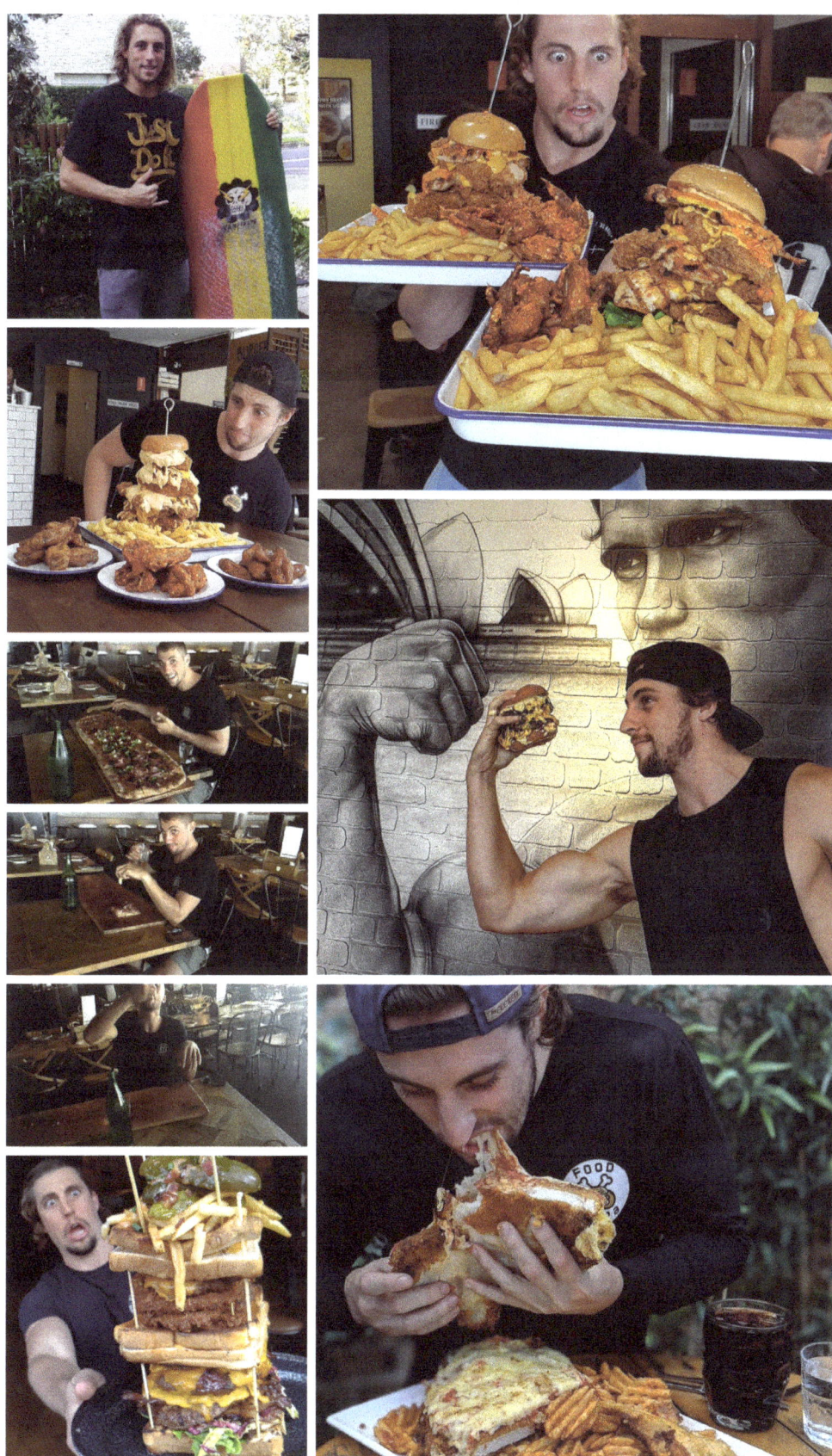

MY TRUE LOVE AND PASSION

In 2017, the burger industry in Sydney was booming and as a result, a lot of my challenges were burger-related. Very quickly, these became popular on my Instagram. People were in awe of the giant cheesy mountains that I'd consume on a weekly basis, so much so that I started to eat them midweek, posting them on my feed. It became my niche. People started to associate me with burgers and became fascinated with all the incredible creations in Sydney. It became my life.

I realized that there was something so special about burgers. I found them to be very freeing; you could add whatever twist you wanted to them and, as long as it was well thought out, it was delicious. You can make a barbecue style burger, with slow cooked smoked meats in there, but also very quickly switch gears and create a fresh Mediterranean style burger with lamb, feta, and hard-hitting spices. In burgers, I had found one of my passions and loves in life.

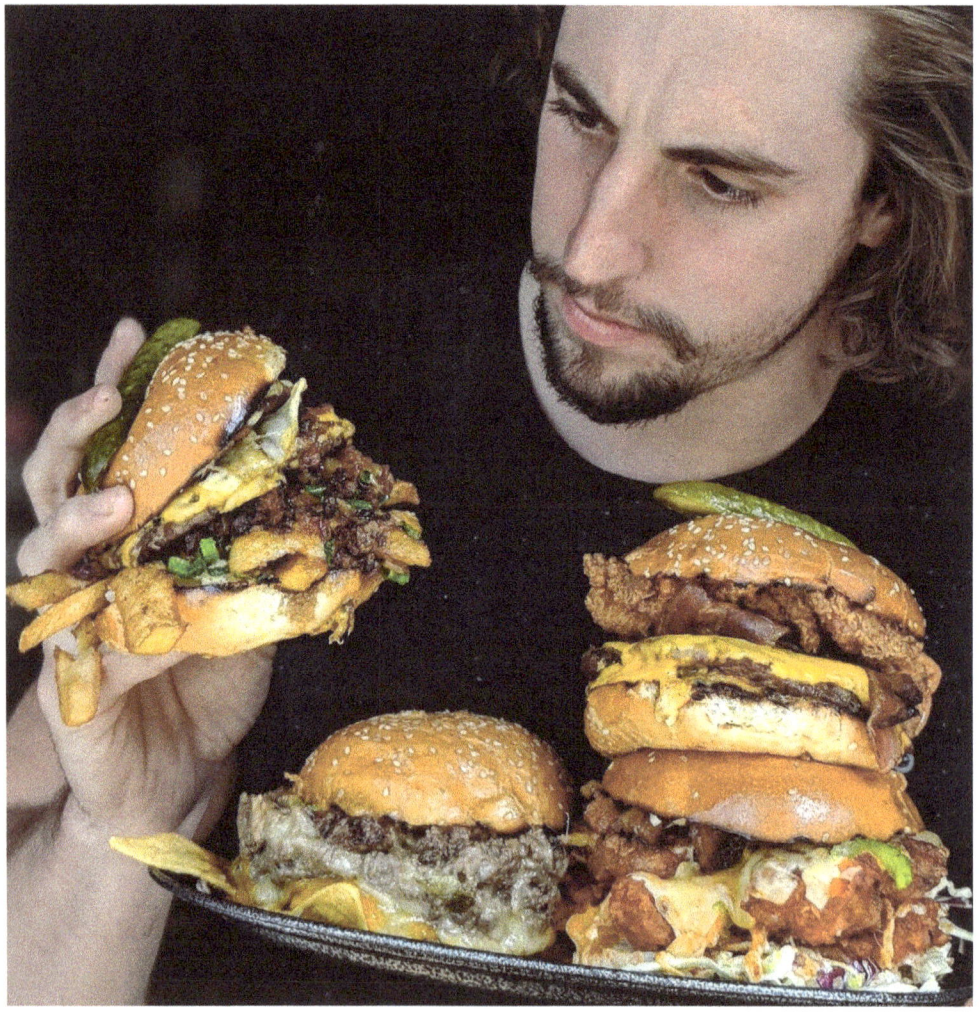

I then met my other passion and love of my life: my wife, Kira. Being the incredibly polite professional that I am, when I first met her, I was her surf coach and, as such, didn't think too much of it. She slowly wore me down with talk of food, the mighty Manly Sea Eagles, and a love for friends and family. Eventually, I couldn't contain my infatuation with her anymore, and I distinctly remember the day I decided to ask her out. I was at a Korean BBQ joint in Chatswood, celebrating my friend Nikki's birthday. At that time, between challenges, I had to consume less food to offset the thousands of calories I was consuming on the weekend. I remember ordering a pathetically small bibimbap. It was polished off in seconds, and I quickly moved on to chat away with my friend, Ella, to distract myself from how hungry I was. The topic of conversation shifted to the cute girl I had been coaching and how I felt unprofessional about potentially asking her out. In classic Ella fashion, she told me I was being an idiot, and to just go for it. And go for it, I did.

Kira then supported me through the biggest transition of my life. I made the move and decided to drop everything to give this food life a real crack. It started with me spending weekdays and weekends out creating content and convincing people to let me help grow their restaurant's Instagram. I missed family events; I missed birthdays; I missed parties, and I missed seeing my friends. But I knew that I had to sacrifice those things I held so dearly in the short term to finally make food my life in the long term. I learned many lessons in the process and slowly but surely built a reputation online and across the food industry. I spent all of my days in kitchens, exploring the world of food with chefs and savoring each piece of information I gained about hospitality.

Eventually, I started to experiment myself. Home cooking became a huge part of my Instagram and my life. I started to put together videos of me slapping burgers together at ridiculous speeds, with adrenaline-inducing music backing them up. People responded massively online, and I received messages daily asking for recipes for my burgers. It seemed like nothing could stop this burger train, and I was ready to take on the world.

Then COVID hit us. Everything came to a screeching halt, and I no longer had the opportunity to grow my business and explore food like I used to. Finally, at the crescendo of my move into the food world, I decided to fill my time by writing this burger cookbook.

And here you are now, hopefully remembering fondly the food that links you to the biggest moments in your life.

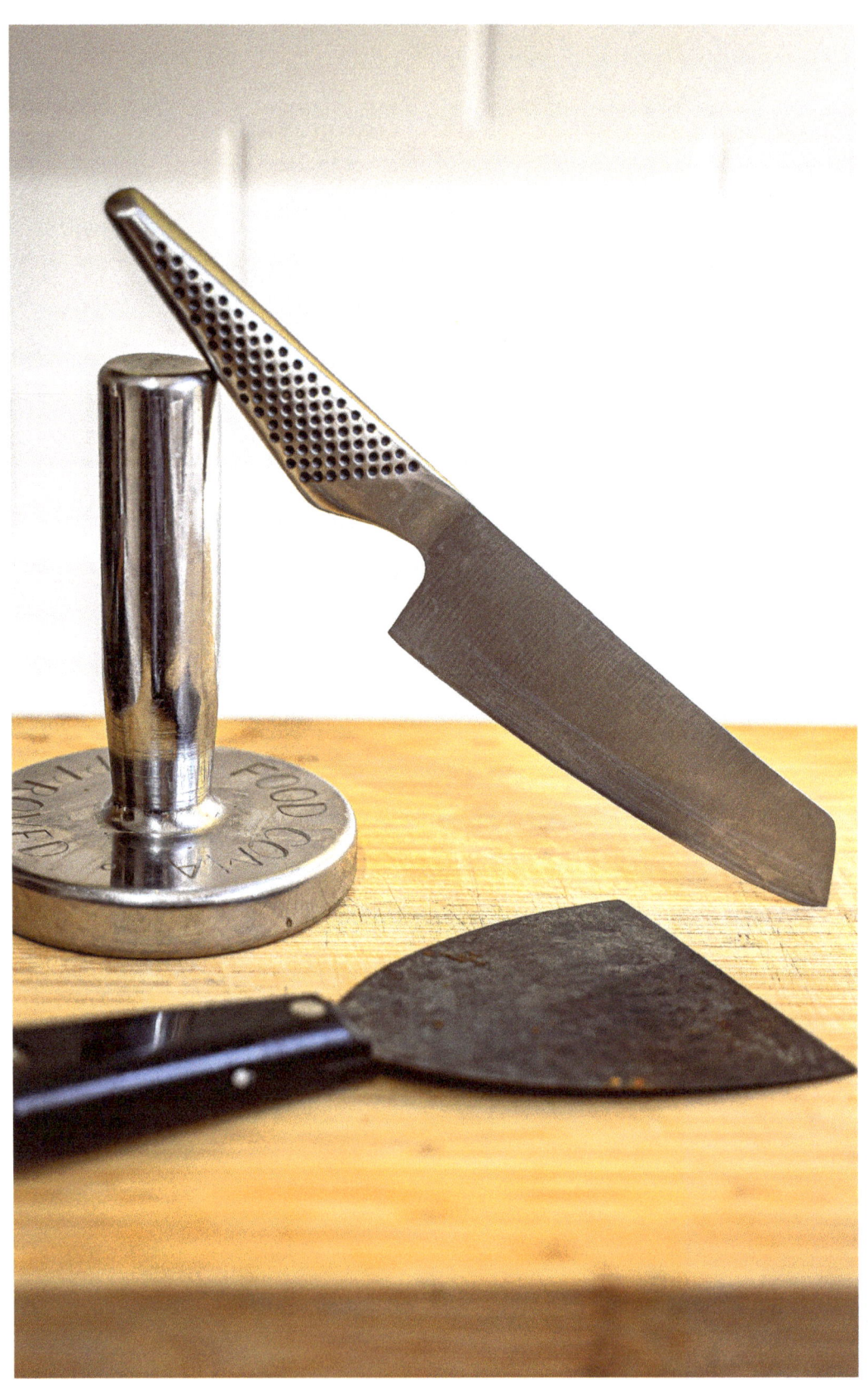

THE TOOLS

Before we start getting into the good stuff (the burger cooking), I feel like it's my duty to help provide some sweet and fast tool/cooking tips for all you budding burger makers. Each recipe may call for the use of a couple different tools, so here's an outline of what you can expect.

THE SMASHER

This cheeky little tool will become an extension of your hand during your burger-making journey. It's your best friend. You will learn to listen to your smasher, feel how it feels, and together you will pound burgers into sweet caramelization. You may prefer a heftier product, or a lighter product, a smaller product, or a larger product. Eventually, you will know exactly what works best for you. Here are some pointers on how to choose your utensil.

THE OG SETUP

Why the OG? Because this is what I started my burger-smashing journey with. Almost every household will contain these two normal utensils, but little do they know the power they have to create ultimate burger deliciousness. Yes, that's right: the humble spatula and a meat hammer (or really anything you can use to press down the spatula). I have no doubt in my mind that you are guaranteed to create just as good a smash burger with this utensil as you would with any of the fancy burger smashers on the market. The catch? You don't look as damn cool as the other guy in your street that has a meat mallet. We all know that guy, the smug bastard with all the bells and whistles. I say this with complete hypocrisy because I've tried almost everything on the market. It was for market research … *Wink*.

THE TRADIE

People look at me with pure disdain when they see my Instagram videos featuring this commonly used tradie tool. Every bloke and his mate have tagged each other laughing, making it well-known—as if it wasn't already well-known—that I'm using a cement trowel to smash my burgers. Well, they can call me MacGyver for all I care; the cement trowel is the *perfect* burger smasher, for a damn cheap price. You can pick up one at any of your local tool shops. They're often stainless steel; they're slippery so they don't stick to your patty; they're just … perfect. If you're handy, you can go a step further— don't hold me accountable for doing this at home, kids—and grind back the metal on the bottom to be a bit smaller and easier to handle. But a normal-size trowel means you can smash out two burgers at once. Pretty handy.

I say this with complete hypocrisy because I've tried almost everything on the market.

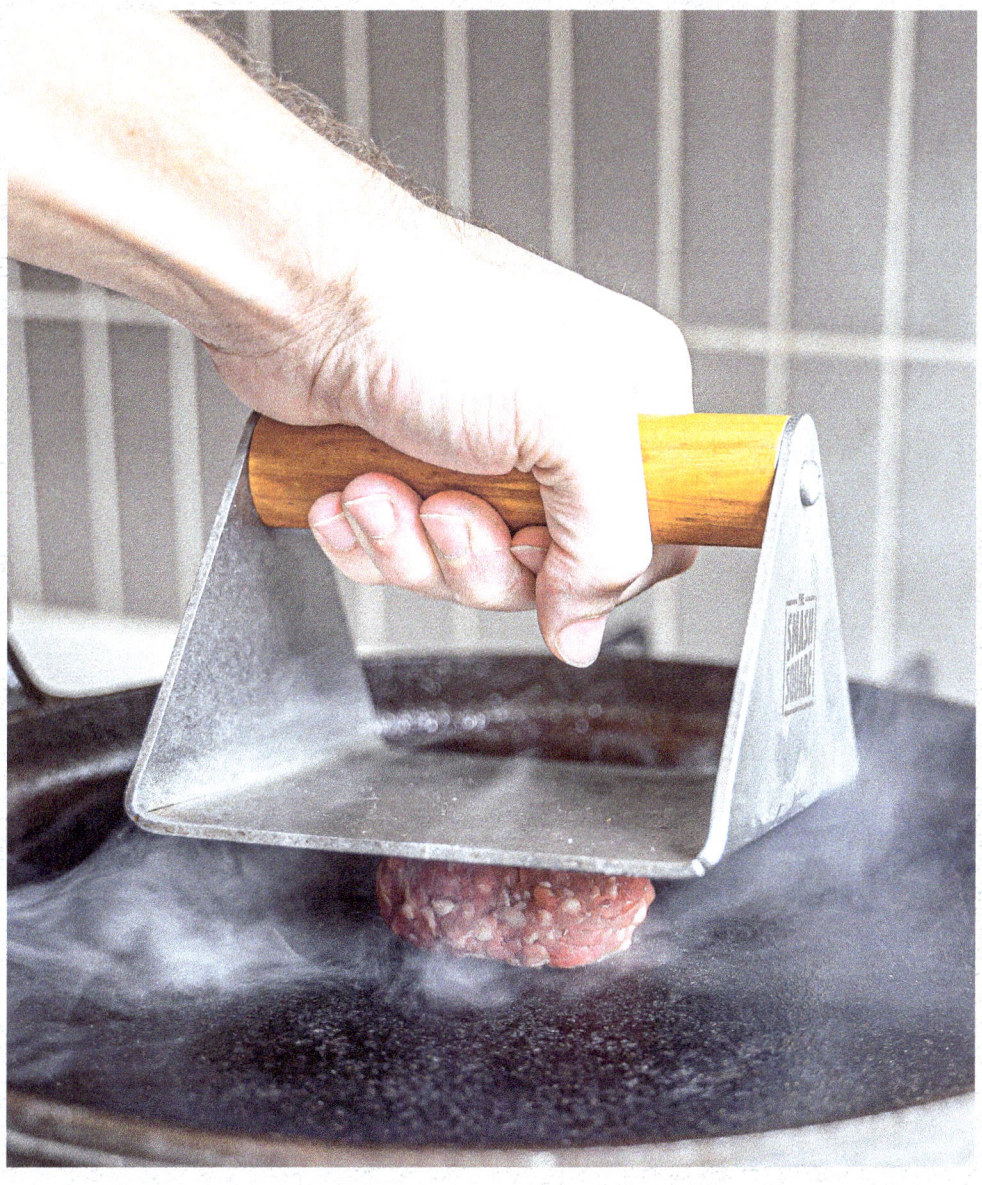

THE SMASH SQUARE

This is not in any way an endorsement. I'm just very chuffed with this one particular product I've tested. In the humble country of New Zealand, a guy reached out to me who was making homemade burger smashers with a similar function to a cement trowel but with a sleek, crisp, and less workman-like vibe to them. It's for the person who can't be bothered to trim down his cement trowel into a smaller size and who finds that the large size can get in the way of smashing on smaller surfaces, like a frying pan. If that's you, this product is perfect because it covers all those bases; *plus* you look really cool holding it in your hand. It's all about appearances, right?

THE MEAT MALLET

Ladies and gentlemen, this is by far the most sought-after product I have ever used in my Instagram career. Every day, without doubt, I have someone approach me asking, "Hey, dude, where can I find that smasher?" However, this is probably the last object I'd use to smash burgers. Yes, I'm serious. Why? Because I feel that you learn the smashing process better when you use one of the above products. And, without a doubt, this technical piece of equipment is the hardest of them all to use. It seems counterintuitive because it looks the coolest; everyone seems to use one, and it's heavy enough to do the work for you. *But!* It often sticks to the patties very easily—unless you warm it up, but then you may overheat it. It also makes a lot of noise when you're pressing the corners of the patty into the grill, and the technique required takes some getting used to. So, do yourself a favor and learn on one of the others, then transition to this piece of equipment as your final stage of burger smashing domination.

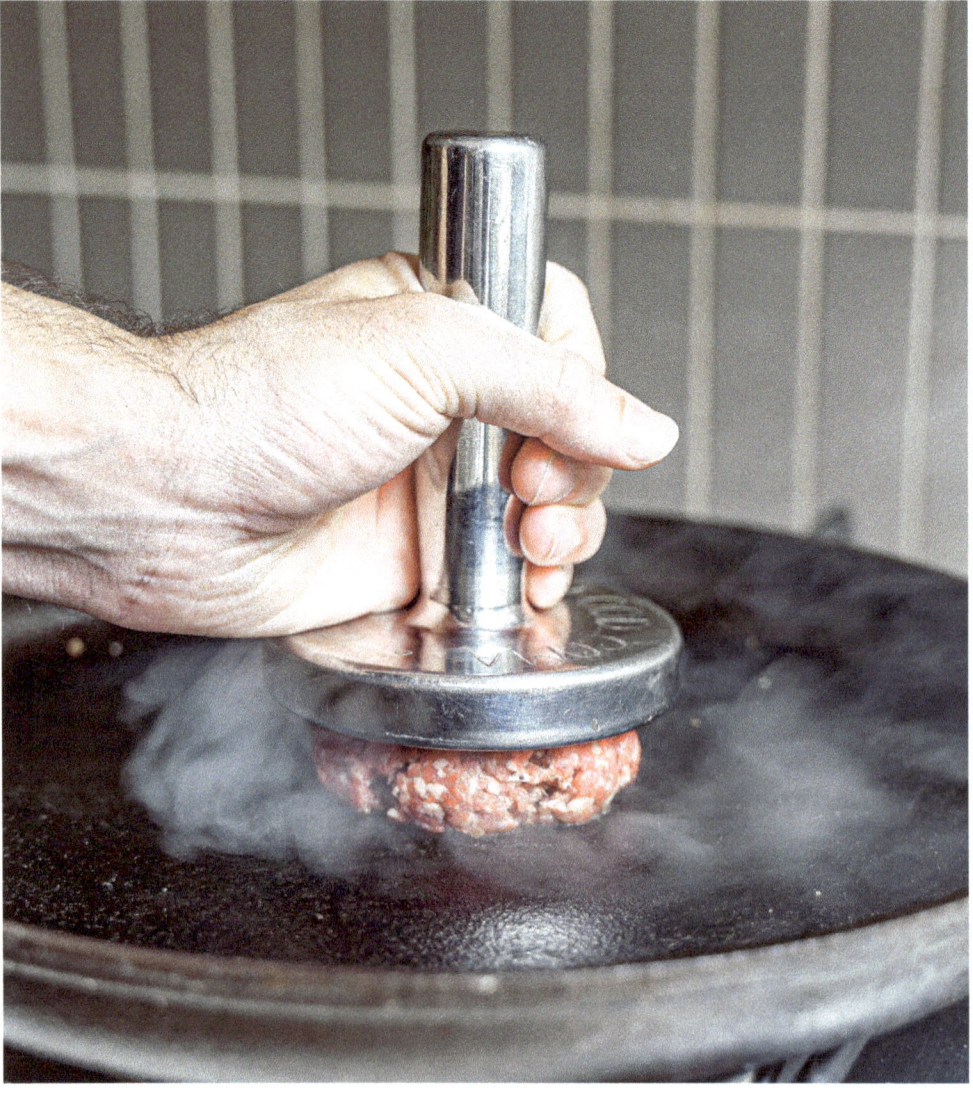

THE GRILL (OR NOT)

It's all well and good for us to have fun looking at what we're going to smash these cheeky fellas with, but you need something to cook it on. Your choice of grill is just as important as the meat, ingredients, utensils, buns, and more. Choosing your grill is a very personal experience. It involves so many factors: how many burgers you're looking to cook at a time, whether you live the apartment life (holla!), whether you have gas or induction in your kitchen, whether you want to delve into chargrilled burgers, how long you're willing to wait for the grill to heat up, and whether you're looking to set yourself up personally or commercially. There are many debates around, and many positives and negatives to, each piece of equipment. Like everything in this book, it's the dealer's choice. You choose your journey. That's the beauty of burgers.

Choice. You choose your journey. That's the beauty of burgers.

THE DAD GRILL

This is not me throwing shade at dads. I can't wait to be a dad one day—poor kid! This is just an observation. I swear on my unflipped burger's life that almost every dad I know has the classic BeefEater/Jumbuck/Traeger/Matador/Weber three to four burner, half chargrill, half flat plate grill. I hope to one day be this guy, but with seven other barbecues. Consistently embarrassing my teenage kids, with my dad bod on full display, as I attempt to crack wise ones while the beautiful aroma of sizzling beef fills the air—the thought brings a smile to my face. These babies are incredibly versatile but can be a little lacking in specialty for smash burgers. Often their flat plate can only fit two to four burgers, depending how thin you smash them and how big the patties are. They can also take a bit of time to heat up and are difficult to clean. The dad grill is a great option for someone who's not a die-hard burger fiend, who enjoys cooking other things, and can tell a whopper of a knock-knock joke.

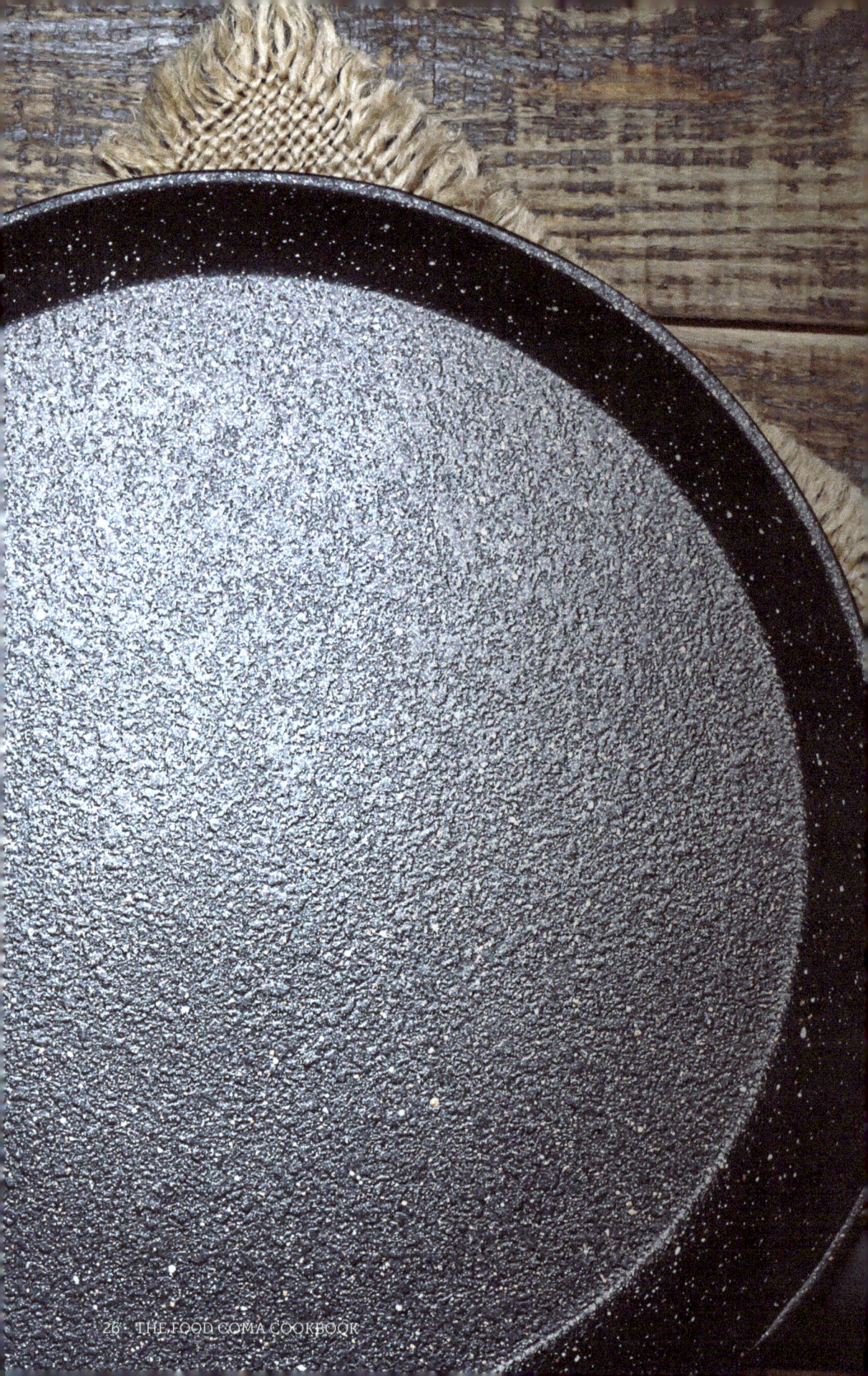

THE ELECTRIC

Living in an apartment has its positives and negatives. You might have noisy upstairs neighbors who always seem to be up too early or too late. You often don't have a sweet backyard for all your toys, barbecues, cars, sports equipment—you get the gist. Space is limited, and it leaves you with only a couple of options. There are two scenarios: you either have a balcony, or you don't. If you do, congratulations! You're lucky enough to have just enough room for *one* toy. Here's one you can choose.

The electric grill isn't the most powerful or versatile piece of equipment, but it can pack a lot of punch for the space it takes up. Often, they range *hugely* in price, anywhere from $250 AUD to $4,000 AUD. The majority of the cost comes down to grill thickness, quality of material, gadgets, heat control, and more. In my personal, completely unprofessional opinion, the $250 product should do you just fine. Grill thickness isn't a huge issue if you're looking to cook only one batch of burgers (generally these will fit around six). The edges of the grill may not be as hot, but if you leave it to heat up enough, it'll get 90 percent of the way there. You can put it on a bench top; you can easily transport it, and it's incredibly easy to take care of. It's a bit of a sterile option; there's not a lot of excitement to it. You can't really brag to your mates about your fully sick countertop electric grill, but it's a no-nonsense, clean and easy way to smash burgers.

THE BIG BERTHA

Alright, we get it. Yes, I'm talking to you, Gary Got All the Gadgets. You have a big, bugger-off backyard grill setup. It has everything, including a built-in TV where you can watch all your favorite sports highlights while you drink beer and smirk to your mates as you say, "I'm thinking of putting in a hot tub soon, too." You have a mini fridge attached to your grill, a mountain of tabletop space, enough meat in your freezer to clog your already-hard arteries, and the mother of all 8–47 burner barbecues with a built-in rotisserie, oven, air fryer, and, for some reason, it recites the bro code on repeat. I am immensely jealous of you. The only reason I go on such a tangent is because I wish I had every single one of those things—except that weird bro code feature. You can do anything. Literally. All I ask is that you invite me over next time and leave the grill on full heat with the hood down until it's smoking hot. Please.

THE SINGLE PATTY PRO PAN

Quite a mouthful, aye? Ode to you who is constrained to using only a frying pan because you can't fit a grill in your place, or the better half says no. You are a true hero because, against all odds, you are still committed to the burger life. You are where almost every single burger lover starts, so stay true to your colors, and you will kick some serious ass.

The humble frying pan is the cornerstone of grilling all things. It isn't flashy; you don't need the most expensive pan in the market, and we are all in the same cheeseburger-making boat. You have a few options here, just please, for everything that is good and delicious in this world, do not smash your burgers on a non-stick. Stick to (pun-intended) either copper-based, stainless steel, or cast iron for your cooking. Obviously, if you're willing to fork out the hefty dollarydoos for a copper-based frying pan, by all means, go for it. But honestly, a seasoned cast iron is a perfect tool for you to use for cooking smash burgers. You need to treat it with respect, so do your research on how to best look after your cast iron. It will be heavy enough that smashing a burger won't throw it around all over the place. It retains heat incredibly well—be careful of the handle—and caramelizes meat absolutely beautifully.

THE SMASH PATTY SPECIALIST

There is one grill that stands above them all in my mind when it comes to smashing burgers. One grill to rule them all, one grill to find them, one grill to bring them all, and, with its heat, caramelize them in the land of burgers where the meat smashes. I hope I don't sound like a blabbering idiot; this is a truly nerdy moment for me to use that as a metaphor. This is the food coma approved product that is, in my humble opinion, the best all-rounder option for the patty-smashing enthusiast: the humble gas four burner flat grill.

There are so many reasons why you'll look like an absolute pro using a beast like this. First of all, it's got an incredibly large flat space, which you don't share with an open chargrill. This means cleaning is easier; the heat is easier to maintain, and you've got so much more room to really lace out the edges of your smash burger. This grill is the bloke who has all the lads around, always has beer in the fridge, has everyone's favorite type of steak, and shouts you a beer at the pub just because he can. It just keeps on giving and giving. You can caramelize almost anything with ease. The temperature quickly rises, and the grill holds heat and reheats as quickly as you can get the next set of patties out of the fridge. This is the king.

THE MEAT

Choosing your meat is like choosing a good car. You need to consider so many different factors about your lifestyle, budget, and time. Sometimes you'll want a cheap and efficient car because you do thousands of kilometers of driving. And when it comes to burgers, you may want a cheap and efficient mince source. However, sometimes you'll need something that's a bit more reliable, like your ute or 4X4. It can get you anywhere and is always going to be good, but it may cost a touch more or be harder to maintain. Like with a car, take time to consider what meat is best for you, your lifestyle, and your budget.

THE TOYOTA COROLLA
(STORE-BOUGHT)

Ah, the Toyota Corolla. This car is truly a classic little runner, but we're here to talk about mince, right? Well, here are some reasons why the car you don't even feign interest in will get you from A to B with no problems, just like the right store-bought mince. I started my burger-smashing journey with no illusion that I knew anything substantial about cooking, and I only had a pedestrian understanding of ingredients, quality, and balance. I knew enough to know the best option was often a butcher's mince, but how much fat, the type of meat used, and the size of patties confused me.

AN ANECDOTAL DETOUR

I've added a quick little TL;DR at the end of this section. The following story is not necessary for cooking burgers, but is more anecdotal. Feel free to skip it if you want to get to the juicy details.

At a young age, I learned a very important lesson about the importance of improving your craft before going for the best available tool or product in your medium. Many people who follow me on Instagram would know I'm incredibly competitive, so much so that I race my fiancé, Kira, in who can scan their items the quickest at the supermarket. It's a trait that has followed me, driven me throughout my life, and helped me become who I am as a person.

We have a story in my family; we call it "Old Sinker." My brother, Luke, was an amazingly talented young athlete; all my siblings were. He was a rower. No, not the kind who wears budgy smugglers and races boats in the surf. The kind who wore skintight "zoot suits" and rowed on a flat river, often the Nepean near Penrith. *Big* difference. But both dressed equally half naked. He had very humble beginnings. He was one of the shortest rowers in the Mosman club, standing just shy of six foot.

And he was always put with this terrible, heavy, unbalanced, and very sinkable boat they called "Old Sinker." Old Sinker was unforgiving, terribly hard to race in, and forced Luke to hone his skills, concentrate heavily on technique, and battle through each day of training. He did this for quite some time.

However, one day he was given the opportunity to race in a completely new, slick, mean, green, fighting machine of a boat. His career took off, and he became one of the best lightweight rowers in Australia, eventually racing in the prestigious Henley Regatta in England. I have no doubt that if he hadn't injured his back, he would be representing Australia in the Olympics. The story doesn't end there.

I, myself, also competed in a sport that required me to be in skintight Lycra, half naked in front of crowds of people. As brothers, we're alike in this way. I was a triathlete. For some reason, one sport wasn't enough for me; I wanted to exhaust myself every day by attempting to be a battler in swimming, cycling, and running. In all honesty, it was probably the best

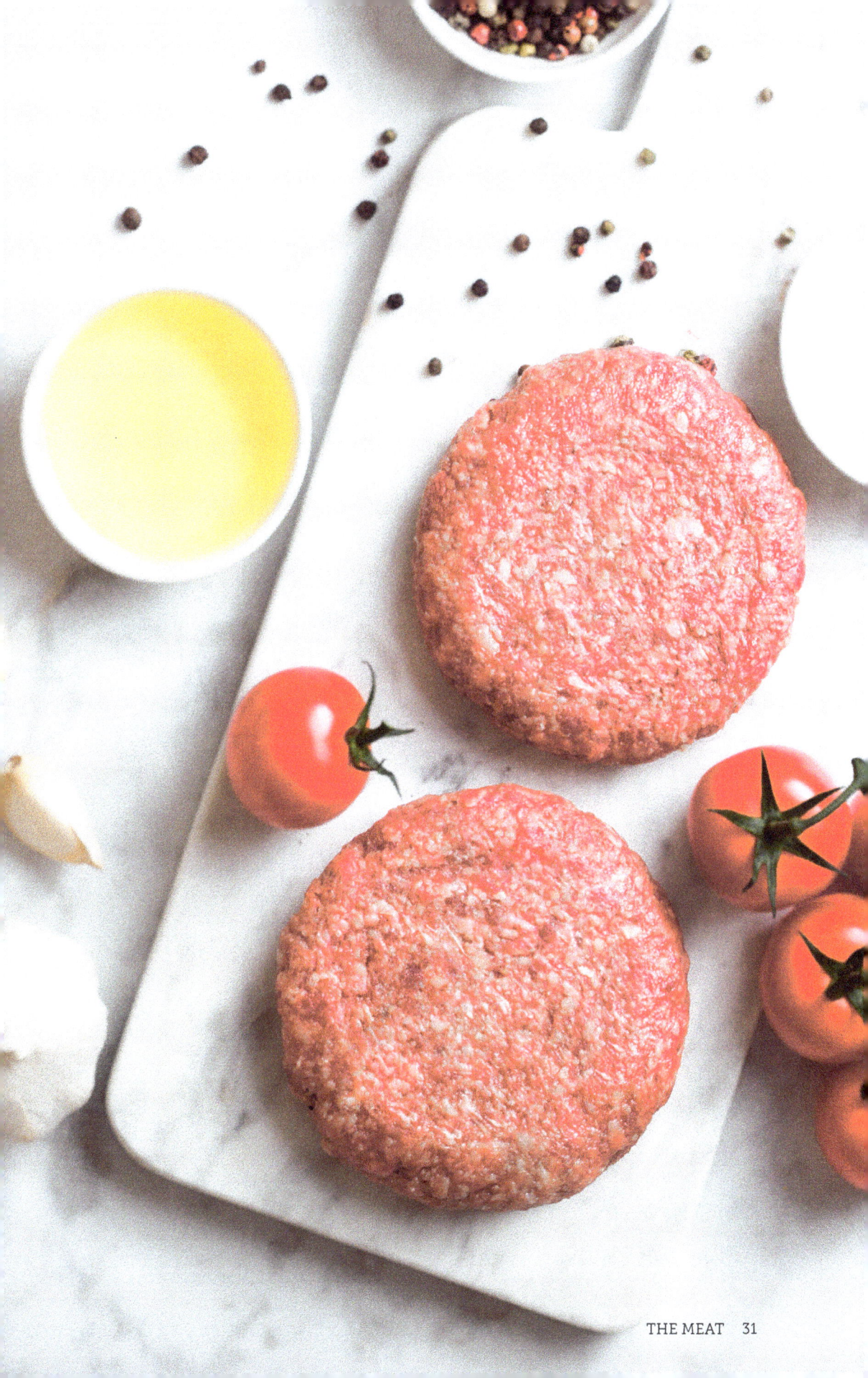

outlet for a young bloke who had self-diagnosed signs of ADHD.

I somehow ended up with my own version of "Old Sinker." It came in the form of a heavyset, terribly geared, unreliable Azzurri racing bike. It was made of a heavier material than most of my peers' bikes, which were often carbon fiber with clinical gearing and worth more than a car. I trained day in, day out on my Old Sinker. Up hills, along windy straights and bumpy roads, and around tight corners. I raced with it and was often modestly placed—nothing incredibly competitive, but enough to be seen as a small threat to the other athletes.

The day I found myself with a carbon fiber bike, there was a ginormous change in the wind. I suddenly went from a middle-pack athlete, a good swimmer who could compete in the bike leg of the race, to one of the best in the state for cycling. The years I had spent on that heavy, horrible piece of machinery had helped me build strength, technique, and endurance under a harder load. In every race, I'd post either the fastest, or one of the fastest, times in my age group for the bike leg and would burn through the competition to put myself at the front of the pack. Too bad I wasn't so good at running!

> **TL;DR**
> If you can learn to be good with crappy things, you'll be even better when you finally make the choice to upgrade.

BACK TO THE TOYOTA COROLLA …

My main point in the above story was to really cement the importance of having a red-hot crack with some of the less impressive equipment and ingredients before you upgrade to the big leagues. I did this with store-bought mince right from the start, and it was very average. But I had the opportunity to learn the intricacies of what affected the taste and texture of this meat before finally giving myself permission to look into custom minces and home-ground patties.

So, have a good go with your humble little Corolla and learn to drive it before getting your hands on a Ferrari. To start, your store-bought mince is cheap and bountiful, like parts for your runaround Corolla. You can very easily pop down to the shops, get your hands on a $5 pack of 20 percent fat mince, and have a quick little burger sesh at home with your friends and family. If you crash your bomb of a Corolla—or mess up cooking your patties—it's not a big deal, and you're not going to be counting every cent the failure cost you. Next thing you know, you'll be whipping your Corolla around the streets comfortably. You'll turn the average supermarket burger mince into delicious, crispy-edged, caramelized goodness and have a ton of fun along the way.

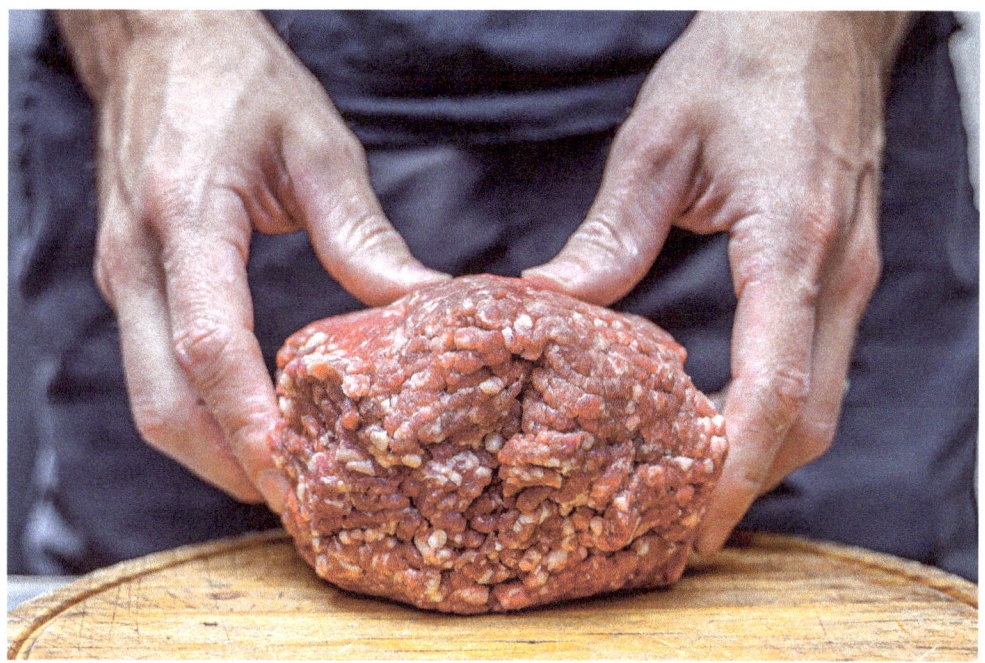

THE 4X4 UTE
(BUTCHER'S MINCE)

How bloody good—sorry, the Aussie in me is really coming out strong now—is a damn ute? Butcher's mince is much like an invincible 4X4 ute that seems to just run forever. You have two options really when it comes to utes and butcher's mince. The first option is to trust the original product made by the manufacturer. Like a ute, you can grab butcher's mince straight out of the window, take it for a spin on your flat grill, and it will be reliably good every time. You can do this for the rest of your life without a worry; she'll always run fine. But there's more to it than that for butcher's mince and utes.

You can customize the hell out of them, and doing so becomes a full-blown hobby and addiction. Fully decking out your 4X4 ute with all the extras, attachments, and upgrades is like getting your butcher to mince a custom patty for you with the meats of your choice. Man, the options are absolutely endless. Depending on your butcher or mechanic, they may love the process of you doing this or absolutely hate the extra hassle. The good thing about custom mincing your patties with the butcher is that it's a much cheaper endeavor than committing to a full 4X4 setup. Head to your butcher, select a few meats, ask them to mince them all together, and often they'll humor you. Then you can start to get a feel for which cuts of meat you prefer to have in a burger patty. You can start basic, using the classic chuck and brisket blend, then move into adding more complex meats, like short ribs (just the meat, not the bone), sirloin, and even adding bacon to your mix. Then you can truly unlock just how cool it is owning a 4X4. I mean, cooking burgers with your own custom mince.

THE FERRARI
(HOME-GROUND MINCE)

I'm not a car expert, but I've heard that Ferrari's are pretty cool. The only problem is they're finely tuned pieces of machinery that require a serious amount of upkeep, can be expensive to own, and need someone who is committed to owning one. When you first start mincing your own patties, it requires an immense amount of practice, can be costly—and technical—and you really need to commit to the practice before you see some serious results.

The first time I ever made my own patties, I was completely delusional, thinking I'd knock it out of the park first go, chest puffed and ego leaking out of my giant head. Boy oh boy, did I get put in my place. At first, everything looked fine. I minced the patties with the coarsest setting; they had a beautiful marbling in them, and I smashed them into the grill, licking my lips and stroking my own ego. It was all running smoothly. The beef was sizzling away, and I watched as the fat leaked away from the patties, and the caramelization started to show. With anticipation and a flair of cockiness, I started to scrape under the patties, ready to unveil a beautiful crust as soon as I flipped the burger. But then, in spectacular fashion, as I quickly flipped the virgin homemade patty, with my face going completely white and an unmanly gasp slipping out of my mouth, the burger turned into Bolognese mince.

It turned out I had made the grind too coarse, and it couldn't bind together. I felt pretty silly. But I gathered up the tattered remains of my ego, which had been scattered all over the ugly-looking scene, and went back to the drawing board. The result? Medium grind. Full stop. I started by doing half finely ground, half coarsely ground, but over the years I've found that the tried-and-true setting for me is a once-through medium grind. As for the cuts of meat I use, I often order a half brisket from Black Forest Smokehouse—they deliver to my door—and just grind down the whole bastard. But, if you want to get slightly more technical, you could add in some chuck and maybe even some short rib. But really, the most important factor here is that you're looking for a higher fat ratio, around 20-30 percent.

Purchasing a grinder to make your own patties should be simple enough. Try not to get bogged down by the large range of products out there. If your main purpose is purely to make burgers, find the cheapest stainless steel grinder on the market and get cracking straight away. I found my first ever mincer at Aldi for $79.99. It did everything I needed it to do and did it well. It was also easy to take apart to clean.

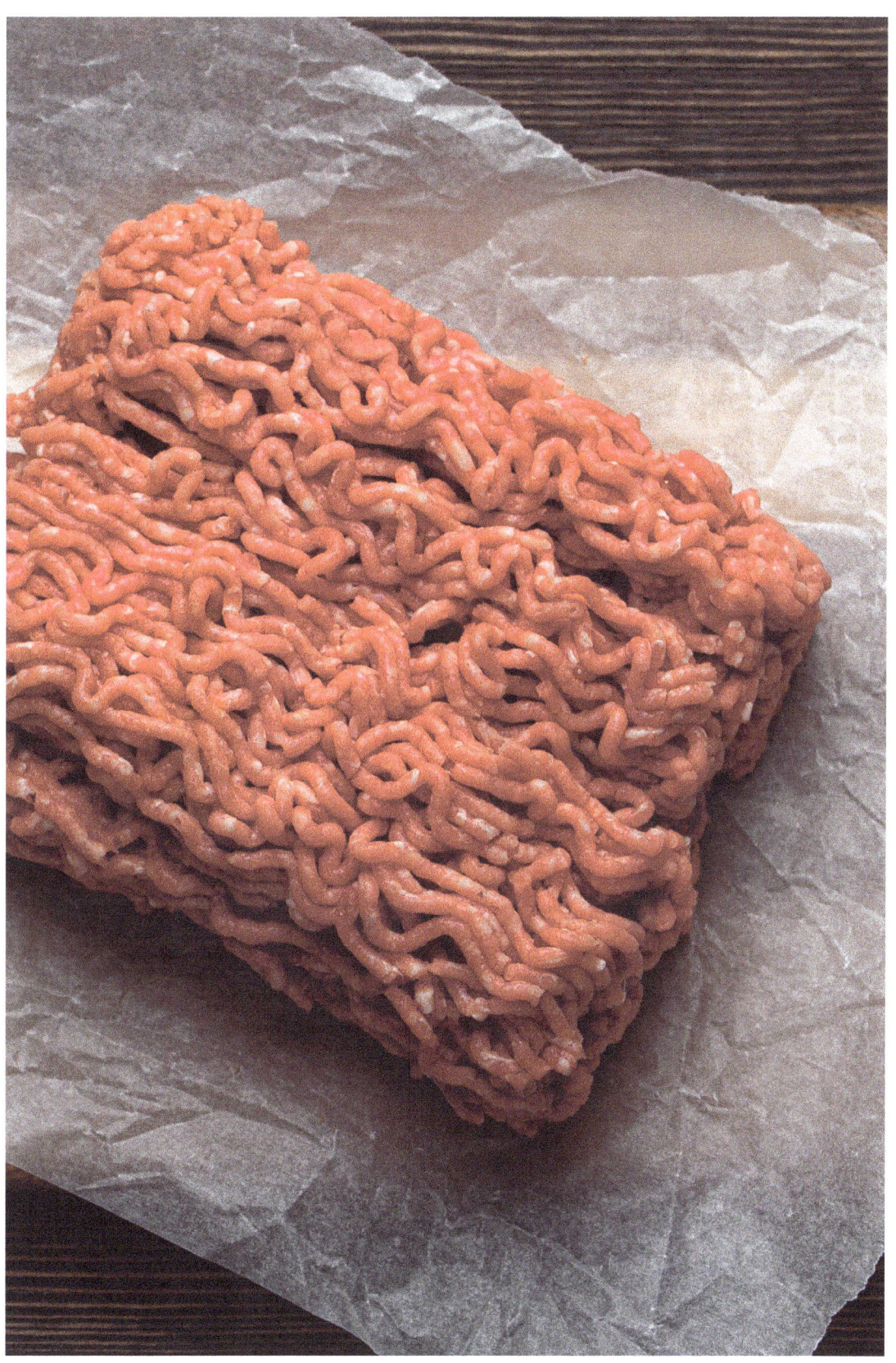

MAKING THE MINCE

When it comes to mincing your own patties, I'm going to try and keep it as simple as possible. Cut your meat into similar sized cubes, 3 cm x 3 cm, and make sure the meat is as cold as possible without being frozen, otherwise the fat smears in the process of grinding. Your grinder can only move so fast, so do your best to not rush the process by clogging up the feed and forcing the meat down with the pressing utensil. One or two cubes at a time until you finish works best.

Make sure you have a nice big bowl to catch all the mince underneath the grinding plate,

One quick pro tip—if you can be bothered, get your hands on a small vacuum sealer.

and flatten it down as the mound starts to heap and fall over. Then all you need to do is massage the mince together so that it binds slightly and weigh out your patties for your burger. One quick pro tip—if you can be bothered, get your hands on a small vacuum sealer so you can store leftover mince for a lot longer and not end up with wastage.

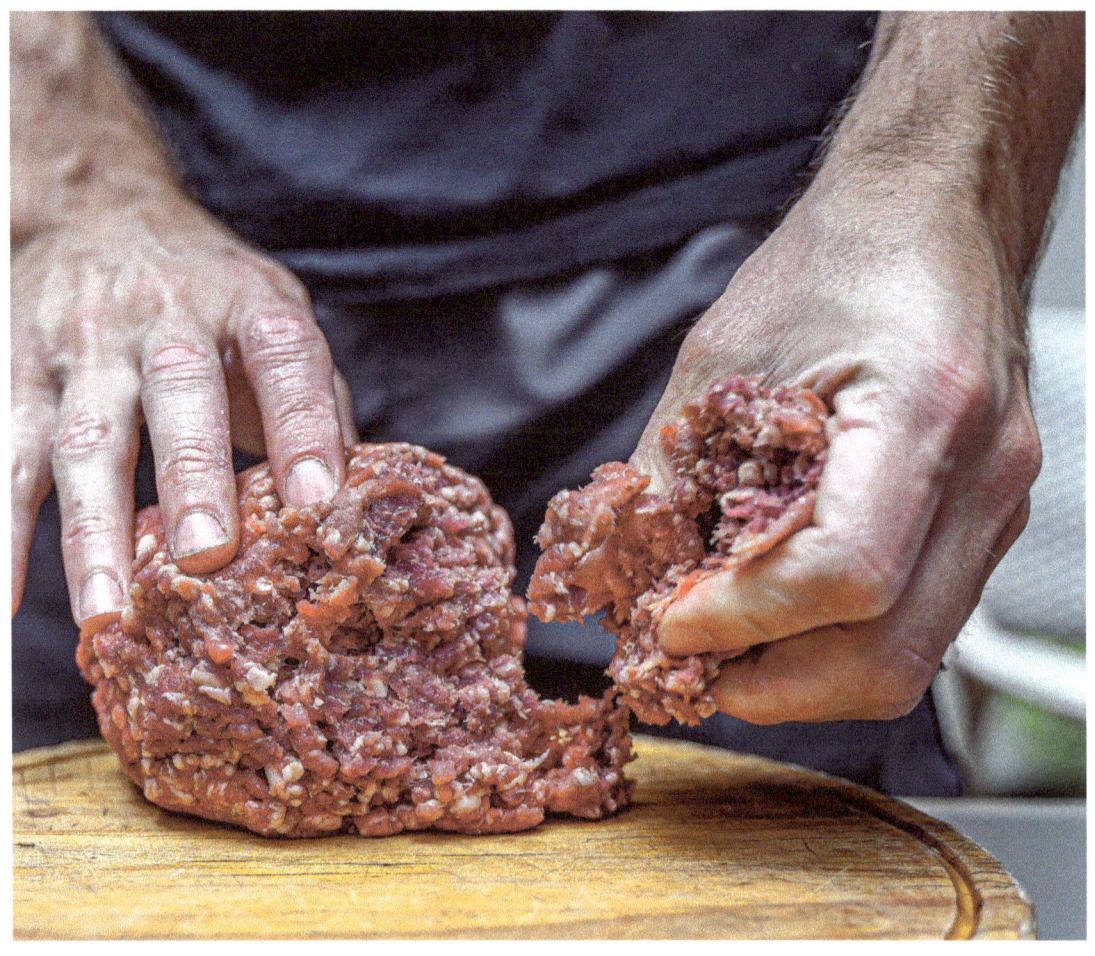

THE SUPPORTING PLAYERS

We've covered nearly everything to get you started smashing those juicy patties, but, like Michael Jordan and the nineties Bulls, you need to give credit to the supporting players as well. These are the tools that you will use for every cook, and each one will make your life easier as you attempt to achieve smash patty stardom.

THE PAINT SCRAPER

No, I'm not and never have been a tradie. I've just found that often tradie tools can be used very effectively in the burger making process. In the famous words of Jake Peralta (how bloody good is Brooklyn 99), "Stuff can be two things." The paint scraper is likely to be the most common tool you will use when cooking a burger. You can use it to clean your grill, scrape under your patties, let patties rest on a colder part of the grill, stack your patties, or even cut bacon in half as you're cooking it. Paint scrapers generally come in varying levels of stiffness, and, personally, I prefer it quite stiff. Hold your laughter in please. This is serious.

The ones that tend to bend more can make it harder to scrape all of that beautiful caramelization off the grill when you are flipping your burgers. They're best suited for those who need a bit of flex because they're cooking on a frying pan and must account for the lip of the pan getting in the way. If you can, avoid getting a scraper that's too sharp. It can strip the grill of some of the protective fats leftover from cooking and if you get that angle even slightly wrong, it can send chills up your spine with a "nails on the chalkboard" kind of feeling.

For those tradies who are rubbing their hands, licking their lips, anticipating cooking some delicious burgers, you cannot reuse your paint scraper for burger cooking. Last I heard, paint is toxic if you ingest it, so put your scraper back in your tool kit and buy a new one. I don't want a lawsuit on my hands.

Process. In the famous words of Jake Peralta (how bloody good is Brooklyn 99), "Stuff can be two things."

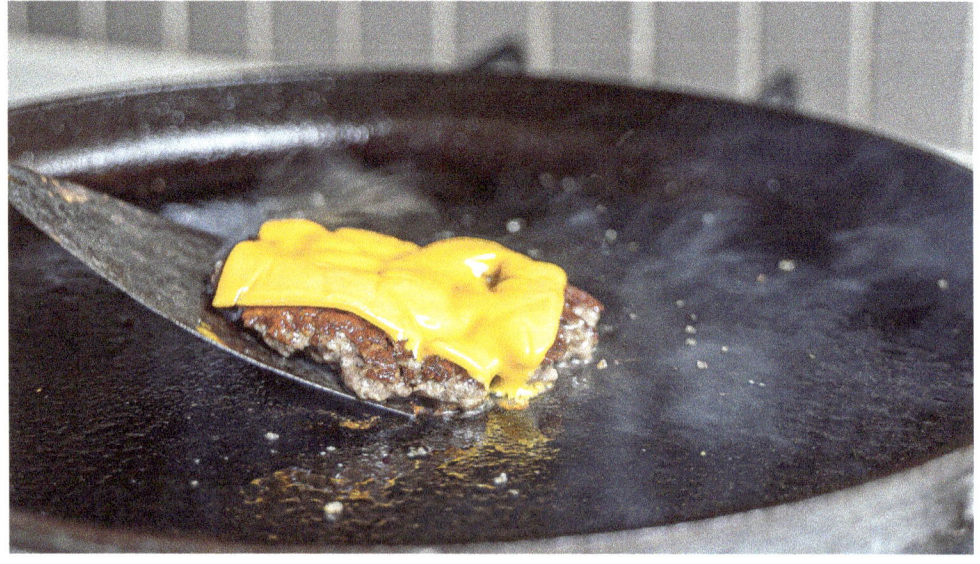

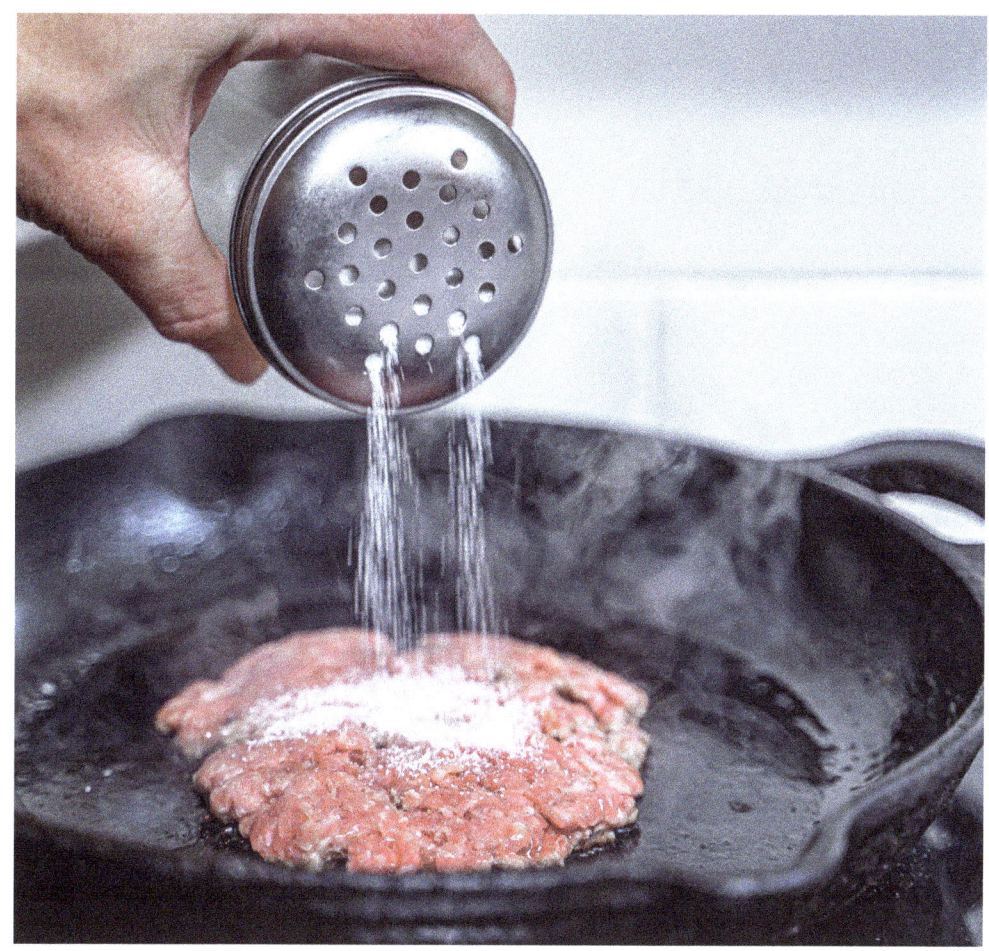

THE SEASONING SHAKER

> *It is the ultimate flavor sprinkler that you can use in all facets of burger, steak, and barbecue cooking.*

Notice how I didn't call it a salt shaker? That's because this piece of equipment can be used for so many more things than just salt. It is the ultimate flavor sprinkler that you can use in all facets of burger, steak, and barbecue cooking. I am genuinely in love with this one cute little aluminum cylinder with holes on top. You could be cooking a mouthwatering, highly marbled, scotch fillet steak with all the Wagyus and Kobes in it, and this little fella right here will help you delicately season it to perfection. A hefty brisket, enough to feed a family of six, or one J-Webby (look the guy up), weighing in at around 5 kg, will need an even coating of seasoning to make sure that beautiful bark comes out crunchy and saliva-inducing to boot. Your burgers, they're like a good beer and can take on so many different flavor profiles thanks to the seasoning you choose to lightly—or heftily—sprinkle over the popping, sizzling beef on your smoking hot grill. Treat this tool with respect. It is your flavor buddy.

THE SUPPORTING PLAYERS

BURGER BUN RUNDOWN

BRIOCHE BUN
The brioche is your go-to bun for many burger creations. It's a sweeter bread than other options but not so much that it feels like you've skipped right to dessert. Brioche buns are ideal for when you want to add a little more oomph and really enhance the good stuff in between.

MILK BUN
The milk bun is soft, airy, and will soak up those juices like a delicious, golden sponge. The bread leans more towards a savory flavor than the brioche does and is great for holding everything together without distracting from the main event in the middle. A great all-rounder!

POTATO BUN
Perhaps not as common as other options, the potato bun adds a slightly different dynamic to your burger creation. As the name suggests, the primary ingredient is potato. The bread can straddle the line between sweet and savory, depending on how it's made, but won't interfere with the between-bun fun. Another great all-rounder if you can get your hands on one.

WHITE BUN
Look, I know that desperate times call for desperate measures, and you may not always have the right type of bun handy when whipping up a burger creation. If you simply must resort to a plain, white bun, you'll get no judgment from me. Actually, I take that back. I'm totally judging right now.

GLUTEN-FREE BUN
I'm going to be brutally honest here: removing the gluten from a bun is like stealing the soul of the burger. Look, I know that some people are gluten intolerant. I get it. If they eat gluten, they're going to have a bad time. But if that's you, I want you to ask yourself... is it not worth it? For those who are genuinely Coeliac, carry on soldier. You do you.

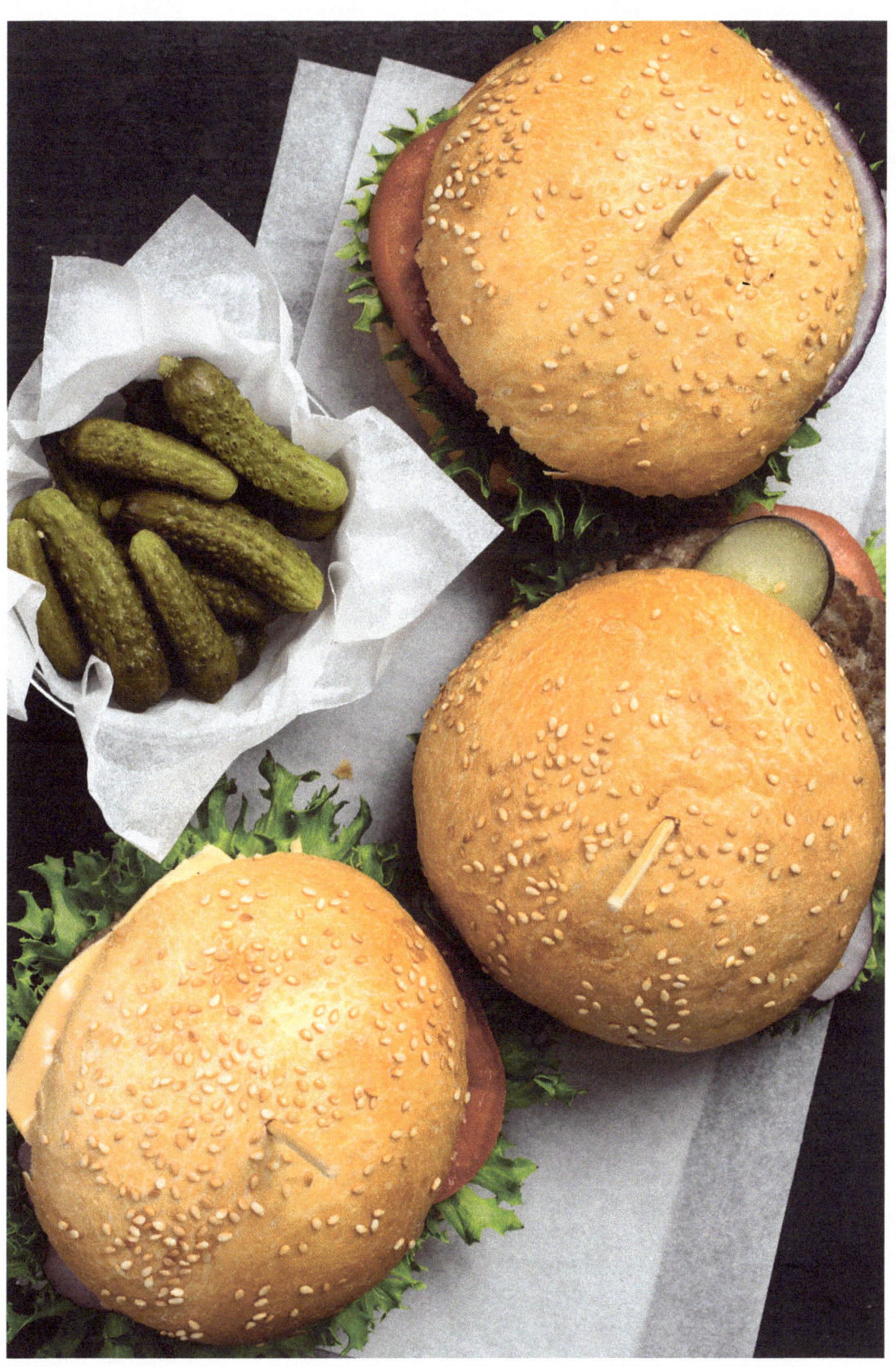

THE BOWLS

For those who just got excited, thinking this is going to be some "420 Blaze it" joke about how one surefire way to enjoy these burgers is to get high, I really do hate to disappoint you. This is as literal as it gets. You need an assortment of bowls, varying in sizes, to help you get the most out of your sauce making and mince mixing. I don't need to go into much detail here. Hopefully, you're all smart enough cookies to work it out.

THE KNIFE

I'm just assuming here that every household has that one knife. It's the knife that has been made famous by both real-life chefs and murderers in movies. I like to call it the "stabby stabby knife." If you're still scratching your head about what I'm talking about, go ahead and google "Halloween knife," and you'll get my point. There's nothing worse than a blunt knife, so make sure you keep yours well sharpened so you can slice through objects swiftly and without any catching. Vegetables and meat, that is. Not people. Don't do that.

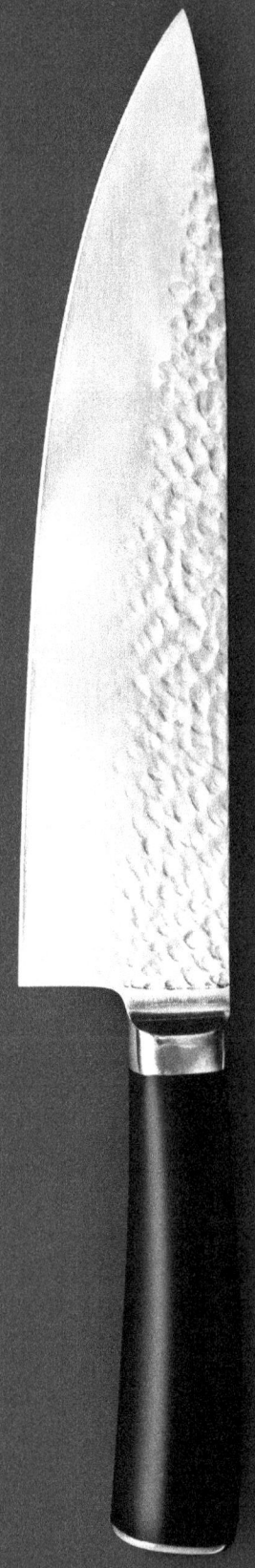

THE SMASHING SYMPHONY

As you get more acquainted with smashing burgers, you'll notice it becomes much less of a brute act, obliterating a patty into a grill with a deep grunt of effort, and more a delicate dance. Time will move in slow motion while you watch as every single grain of patty is laced out on the grill in front of you, each individually grilling away in a perfect symphony. Your final prize will be a meat that's brown and crunchy on the exterior, yearning to be placed between two buns and paired with a homemade burger sauce. Or not, maybe that's just me. There are two styles I like to use when smashing patties, and each has its own advantage over the other.

THE FLAT SMASH

This is by far the easiest smash to perfect and, sadly, a lot harder to do with the meat mallet. First of all, you'll want to weigh your patties to the desired size. Generally, for a flat smash, you can venture anywhere from 80 g to 150 g patties. The main difference between the two will be how thin you smash it down. The smaller the patty, the thinner it will be, and the quicker it's going to cook. When you're working with a big 150 g fella, it will be a lot thicker, but you'll be smashing it out to about the same width.

You'll want to have those patties slightly dry and relatively cold. The best way to achieve this is to throw the suckers in the fridge for about ten minutes before cooking. You're probably wondering why on earth that makes a difference. Well, listen closely buddy, friend, guy—it makes a *huge* difference. A cold, dry patty won't stick to your smashing utensil and believe me when I say that it will save you a *lot* of hassle. Also, you'll avoid uttering unmentionable words of frustration in front of your loved ones.

Before you start any sort of cooking, you want that grill literally smoking hot, so give it time to heat up. This is one thing you really cannot rush. If you're cooking inside, make sure you have the extractor (thing above your stove) on full pelt. You don't want to be that guy who ends up having the fire brigade called on him. The next step is to give your little buddy (smasher) a warm welcome to the grill. To quote a Mike Tyson meme, "Now kith."

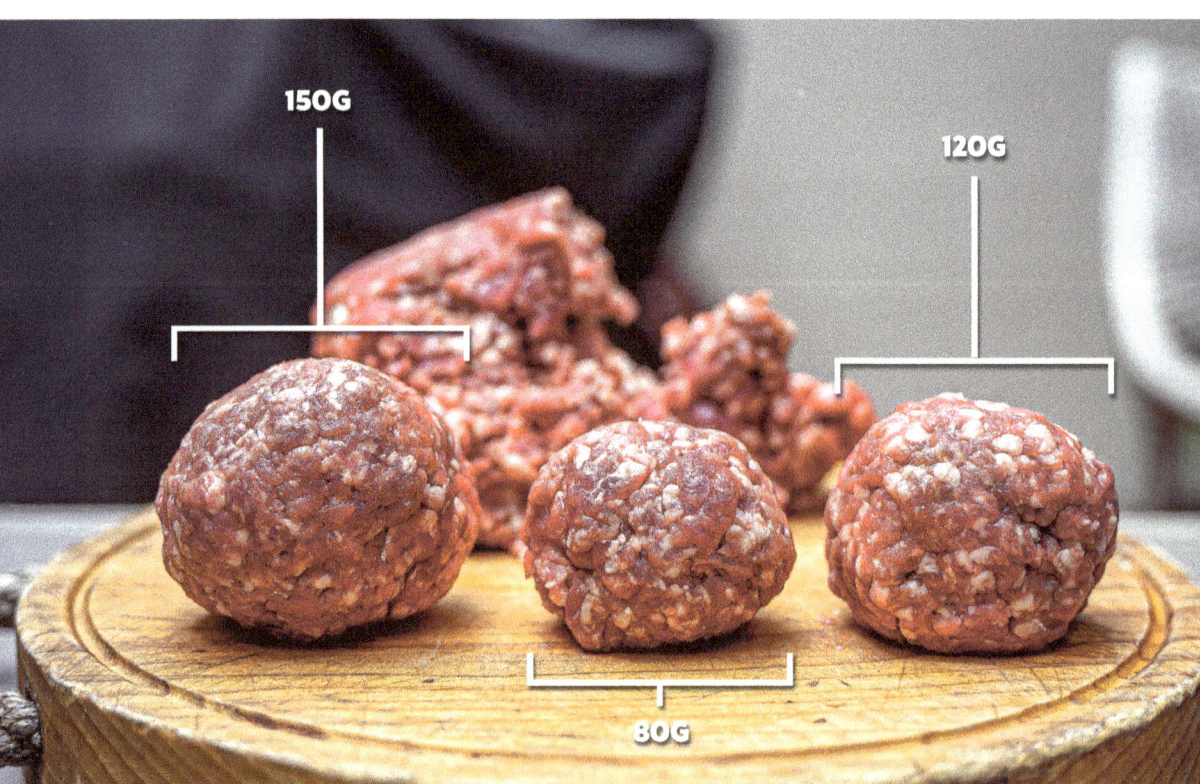

SMASH TIME!

Kiss the smasher and the grill together, rub them for a quick little spell, and they'll both be ready for the smashing. The flat smash starts out simple, exactly like any other. An even ball of deliciously marbled beef is placed on a smoking hot grill or frying pan. Once you've placed all the required balls of yummy on the grill, it's time to start smashing them down.

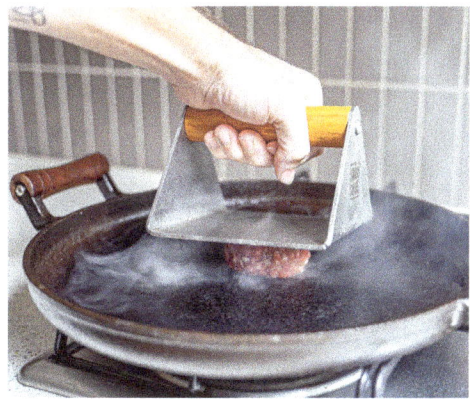

One by one, slowly place your smasher onto each patty and apply even downward pressure, twisting the smasher side to side (to avoid sticking) until the patty is uniformly laid out on the grill. All of the patties should be the same thickness: about 1 cm wider than your burger bun. Remove your smasher, season evenly across the patty, and wait until most of the pink on top has disappeared.

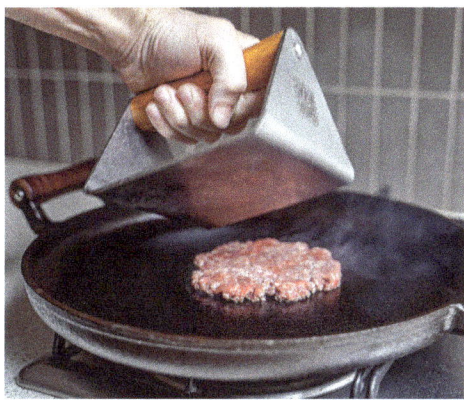

Then grab your paint scraper—minus the paint—and in a small to-and-fro motion, with plenty of pressure applied toward the grill, strip all of that amazing, caramelized beef off the grill until there are no bits remaining. Flip your juicy friend (patty) and quickly put your favorite cheese on top (I prefer hi melt). As soon as the cheese has melted, the patty has finished cooking, and you can remove it or stack it on other patties.

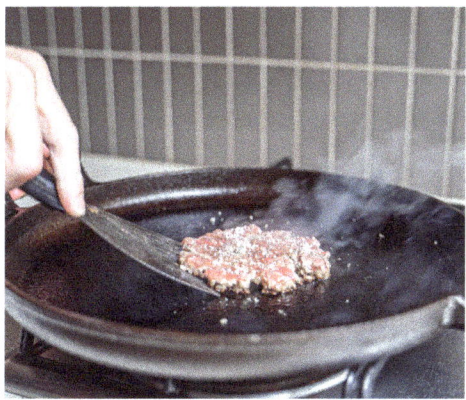

There are two main reasons to choose a flat smash over an edged smash. Firstly, it's much less difficult to master, and you'll be able to quickly smash one patty after the next. It's much easier to punch out when you've got multiple burgers to cook. Secondly, the patty cooks more evenly and a touch slower than your edged smash, giving you a more consistent and

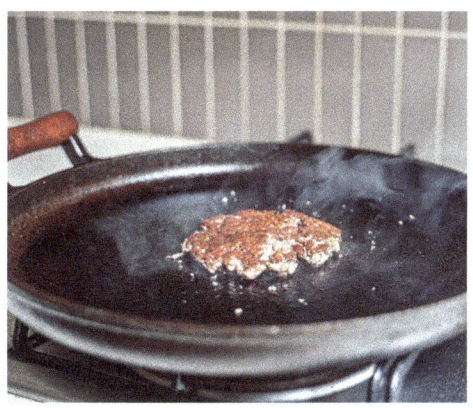

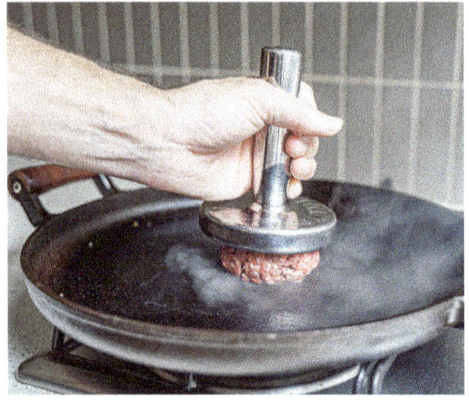

easier mouthwatering product. However, you don't look as cool doing an edged smash, so what's even the point?

THE EDGED SMASH

I'll be honest: the edged smash looks, tastes, and feels awesome from start to finish. You feel like an absolute pro when the smashed-out beef starts to curl up and become a lacy tapestry of caramelized goodness. It creates a beautiful crispy edge that adds to the texture of any burger, with a juicy center to complement it.

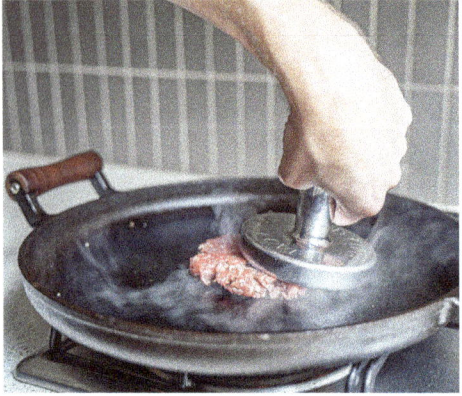

To do an edged smash, follow all the steps above until you start to press down your patties. For this one, you want to alter your technique slightly. Instead of pressing the patty down flat until it's about 1 cm wider than your bun, you want to smash it down to just shy of the bun width—and here's where the magic happens. From there, you want to massage the edges of the burger into the grill, pressing them until they're nearly paper-thin, while keeping that center approximately 1.5 cm thick. From here, it's the same process as any burger. Season, flip, cheese, melt, remove/stack, and hopefully you'll have a delicious product to put with your bun and assorted condiments.

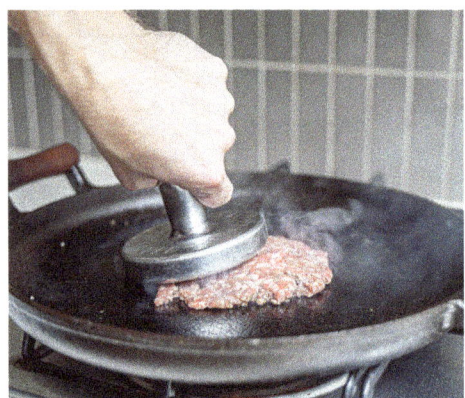

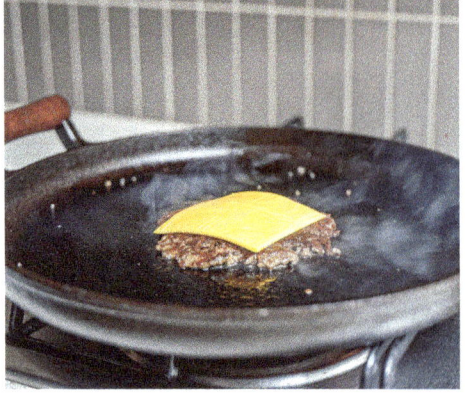

46   THE FOOD COMA COOKBOOK

THE JOURNEY BEGINS

You're ready. I hope you're as excited as a kid on Christmas day, because it's time to get cooking. Remember that Rome wasn't built in a day. If it's frustrating or doesn't seem to be working, step back, take a breather, and have another crack. All the more simple recipes will be at the start of this book, and as we progress, they will become more wacky and crazy. Good luck, I'll see you on the other side.

THE OG

Like every good restaurant, you need a heavy-hitting item that almost everyone will enjoy, something you can whip together quickly on the grill for several hungry bellies. A burger so easy, you can smash out a few cheeky fella's while it's halftime in your favorite sport. I'm going to show you just why this burger is possibly the best in this recipe book. All you need are high-quality ingredients, a strong proficiency in smashing burgs, and a hungry herd ready to enjoy your product.

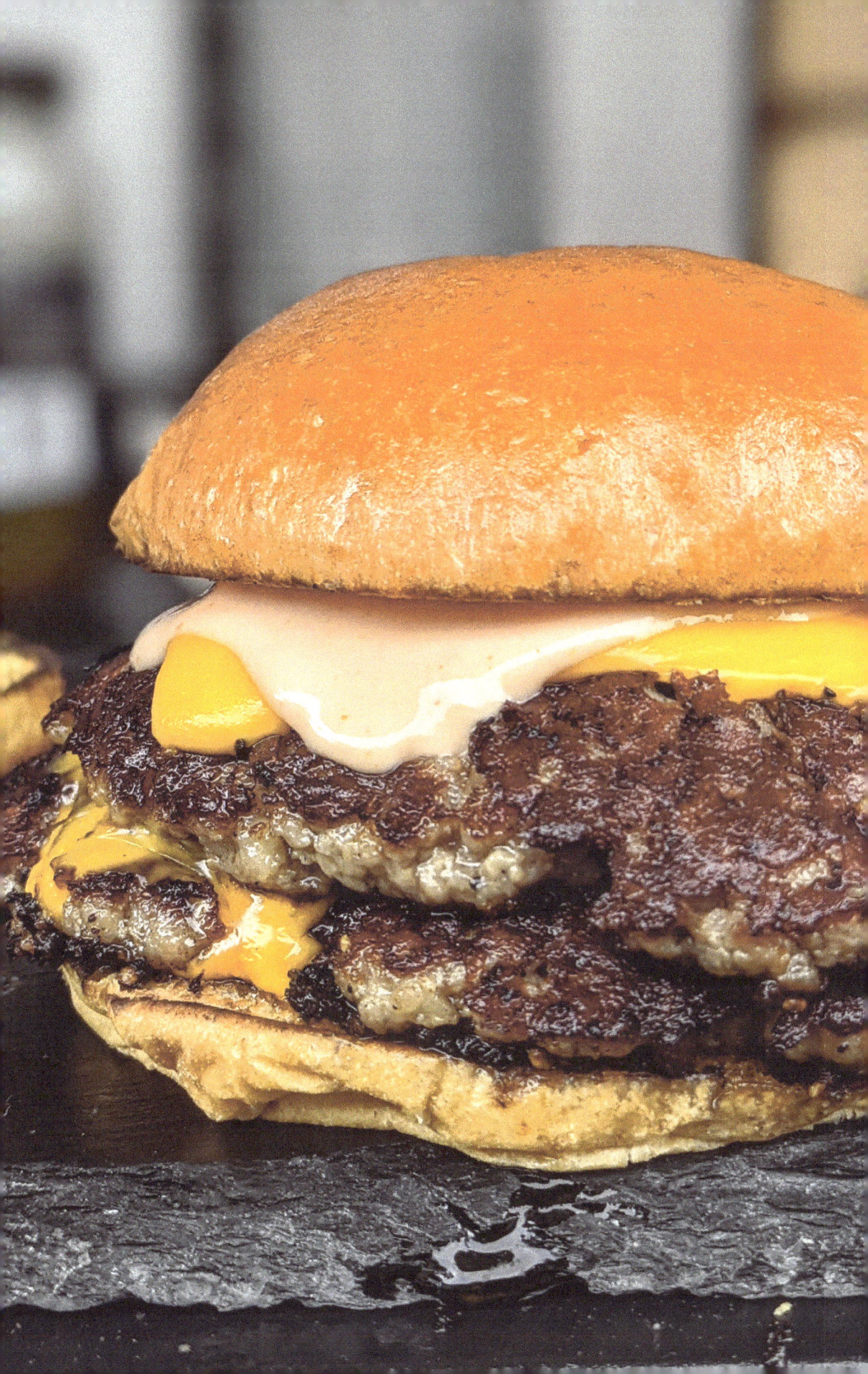

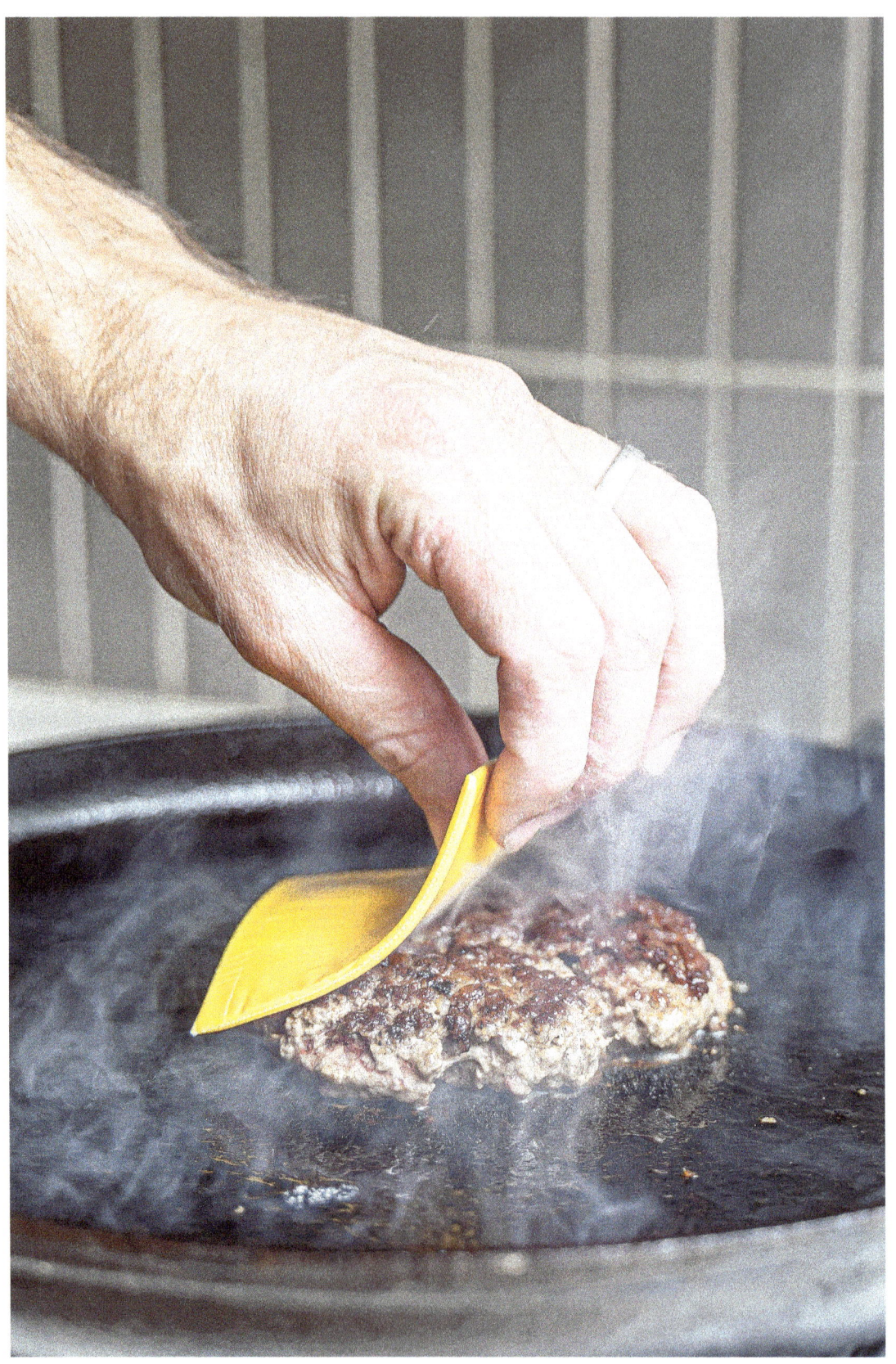

THE SAUCE

60 g of whole egg mayonnaise
40 g of ketchup
20 ml of sweet pickle juice

Start by creating your sauce. Put all the ingredients together and mix with a spoon until smooth and creamy. This part of the recipe is discretional, and you can interchange the ingredients at different ratios to your preference. Once mixed, store it in the fridge.

THE BURGER

1–3 x 120 g balls of beef mince
1–3 slices of American hi melt cheese
Sweet pickles
Soft milk or brioche bun
Salt flakes

Prepare your beef into equally sized balls, using either store-bought, butcher's, or homemade mince. Place in the fridge uncovered for 10 minutes prior to cooking.

Cut your milk or brioche bun in half.

Preheat your grill, giving it a good clean with your paint scraper and vegetable or canola oil. Before the grill is at full heat, place the inside of your cut buns on the grill, placing a small amount of pressure on them. Wait until they become soft and airy, and slightly brown on the inside. Remove and put aside for assembly.

Wait until the grill is smoking hot and place your patties on the grill one by one, leaving space between them to be flattened out.

Using your preferred smashing tool—you can either opt for a flat smash or an edged smash—press down your patties to just wider than your bun width. Season evenly across the patties and wait until the pink has nearly disappeared from the top. Flip your patties and place your hi melt American cheese on top of the cooked/brown side. As soon as the cheese is melted, you can remove the patties from the grill and prepare to assemble your burger.

Assemble your burger, placing your cooked beef on the bottom bun, then apply as many pickles and as much sauce as you prefer. I generally opt for 1 tablespoon of sauce and 3–4 pickles, depending on size.

Eat and enjoy!

THE OKLAHOMA STYLE SMASH

I did not invent this burger, nor have I made it famous. This amazing, delicious burger was created by the one and only George Motz. It is a truly tasty and unique burger that hits every spot you could imagine. I believe that every burger cookbook needs to incorporate this creation in its arsenal. Get ready to be blown away by flavor. This is as simple and good as it gets for me.

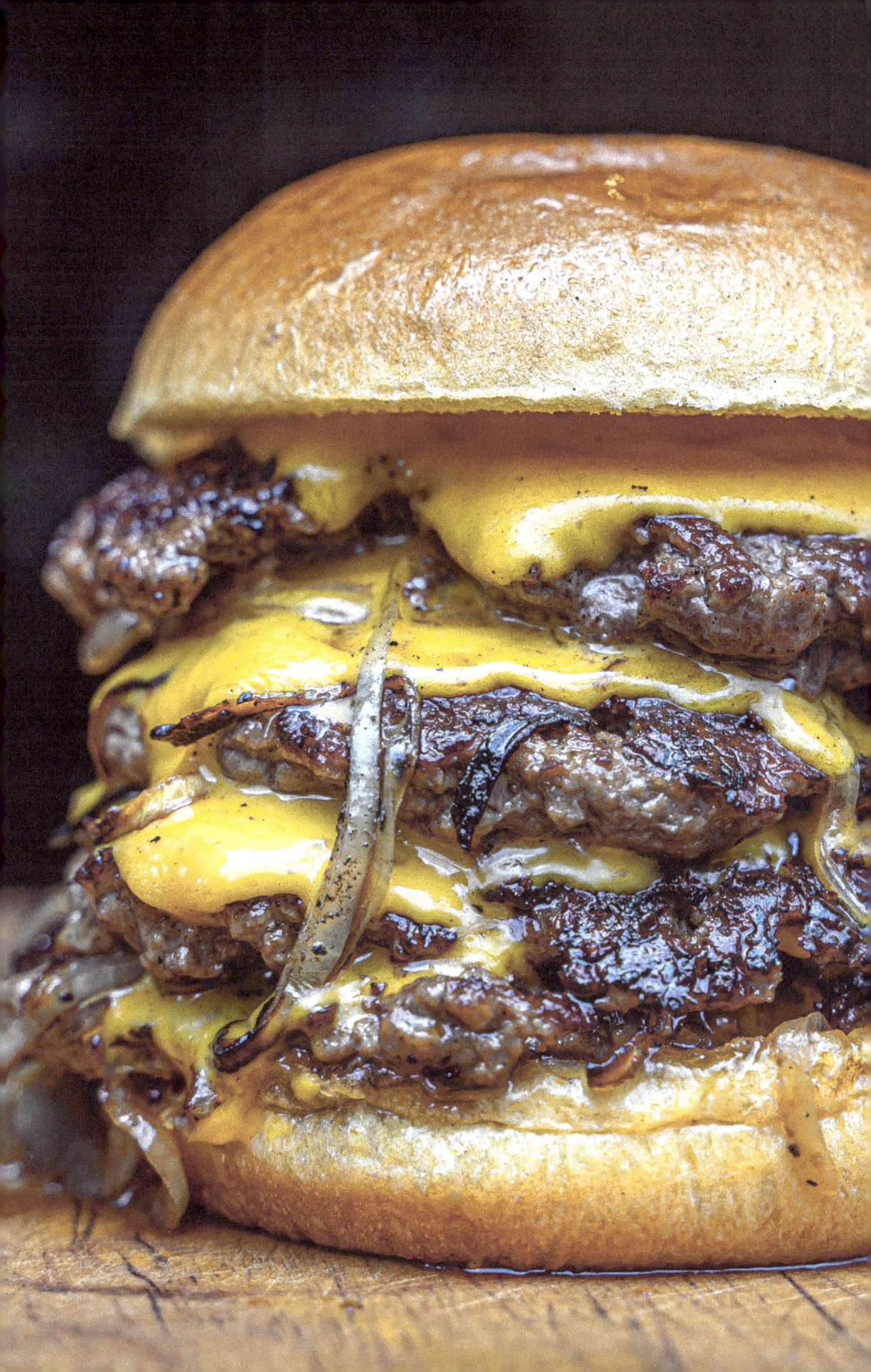

THE BURGER

1–3 x 120 g balls of beef mince

1–3 slices of American hi melt cheese

1 large onion

1 brioche or milk bun

Prepare your beef into equally sized balls, using either store-bought, butcher's, or homemade mince. Place in the fridge uncovered for 10 minutes prior to cooking

Peel your onion, cut it in half from the top or bottom end, and thinly slice the onion into shaved portions, almost so thin you can see through them. Set aside 1–3 medium-sized handfuls of sliced onion to be placed on the patties when cooking.

Cut your milk or brioche bun in half.

Preheat your grill, giving it a good clean with your paint scraper and vegetable or canola oil. Before the grill is at full heat, place the inside of your cut buns on the grill, placing a small amount of pressure on them. Wait until they become soft and airy, and slightly brown on the inside. Remove and put aside for later.

Wait until the grill is smoking hot and place your patties on the grill one by one, leaving space between them to be flattened out. Place the sliced onion on top of these patties.

Using your preferred smashing tool—you can either opt for a flat smash or an edged smash—press down your patties and onion to just wider than your bun width. Season evenly across the patties and wait until the pink has nearly disappeared from the top. Flip your patties and place your hi melt American cheese on top of the cooked/brown side. Lastly, place your top bun on one of the patties while you wait for the cheese to melt. As soon as the cheese is melted, stack the patties on top of each other, with the top bun and patty on top, then remove from the grill and place on the bottom bun.

Eat and enjoy!

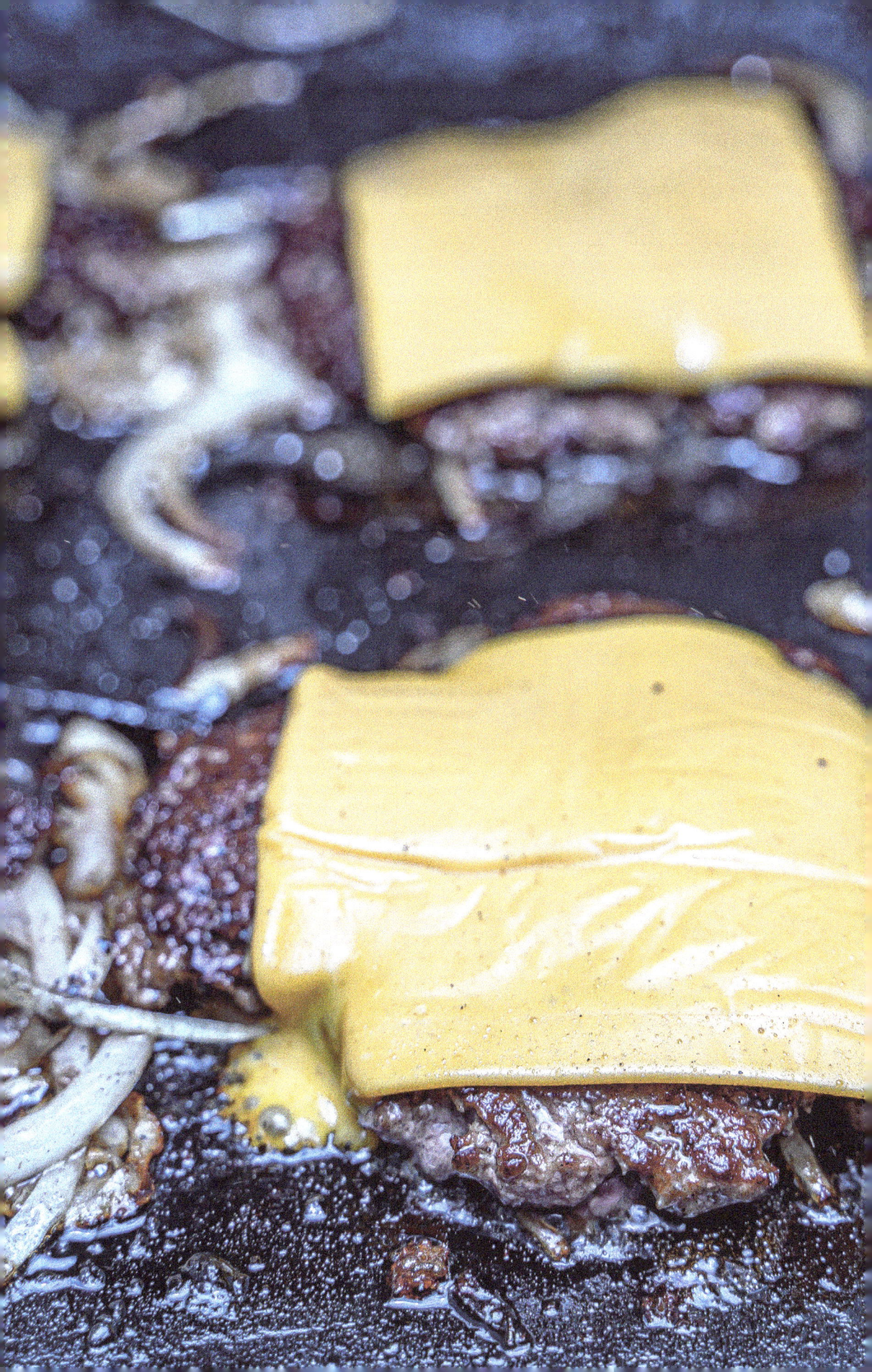

THE HOMER SIMPSON

I want to preface by stating that this is not an original concept by me. This is an already established way of eating burgers that is popular across Australia, America, and many other countries. But, just like the Oklahoma smash burger, it is something I cannot in good conscience leave out of a burger recipe book. As much as I want to show original ideas in this book, I also want to open your eyes to some of the amazing, eye-popping creations from around the world. I will say this: you can use whatever donut you feel is right for you, although I'd go with the original glazed.

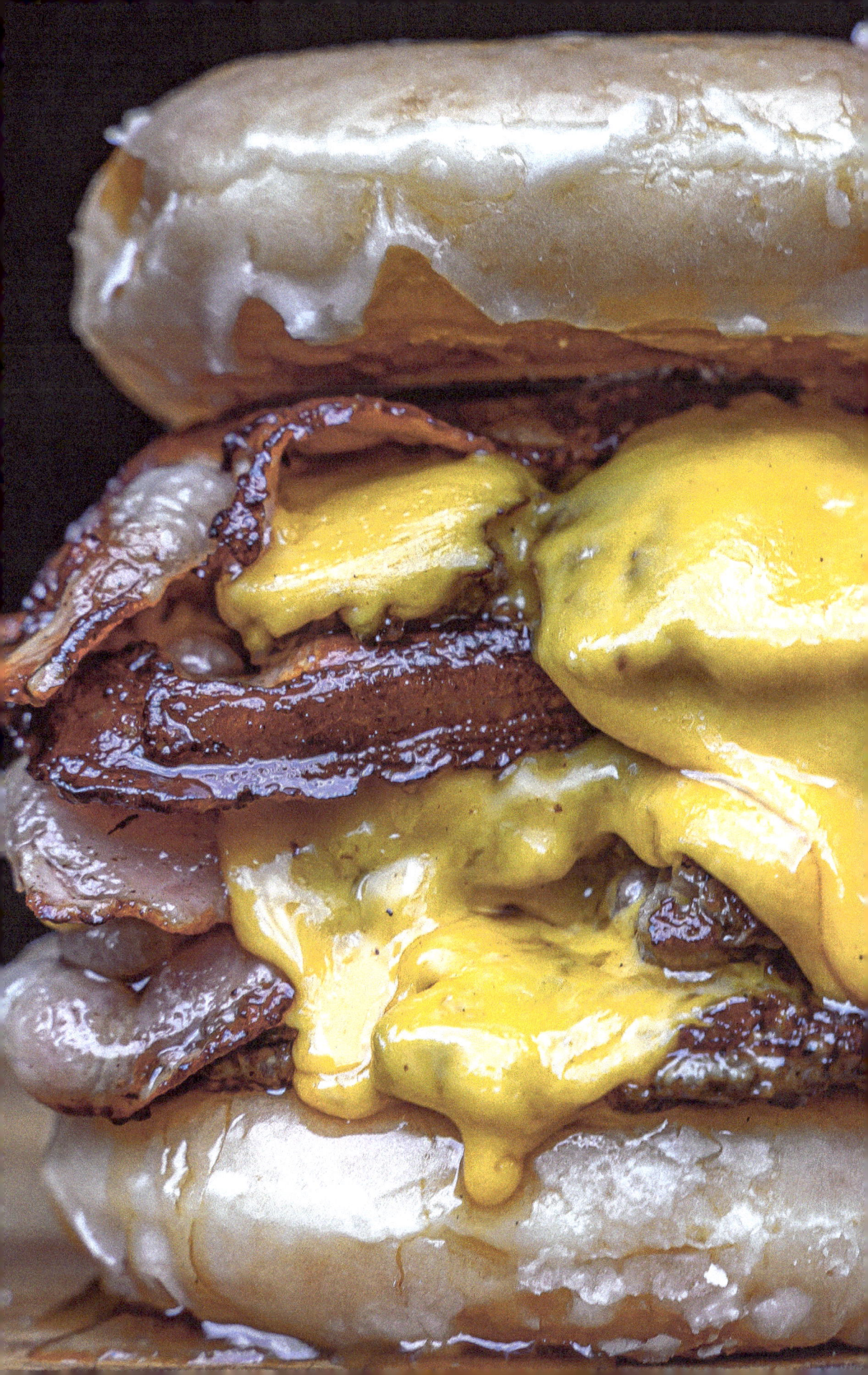

THE SAUCE

60 g of whole egg mayonnaise

30 g of mild American mustard (I like French's)

20 g of ketchup

20 g of Sweet Baby Ray's buffalo wing sauce (or a similar alternative)

40 ml of dill pickle juice

1 dill pickle (diced)

Start by preparing your sauce. Finely dice your dill pickle until it's in 2–3 mm cubes and place it in a small mixing bowl with the other sauce ingredients. Mix them together with a spoon until the sauce is smooth and consistent in color, with bits of the diced pickle distributed evenly throughout.

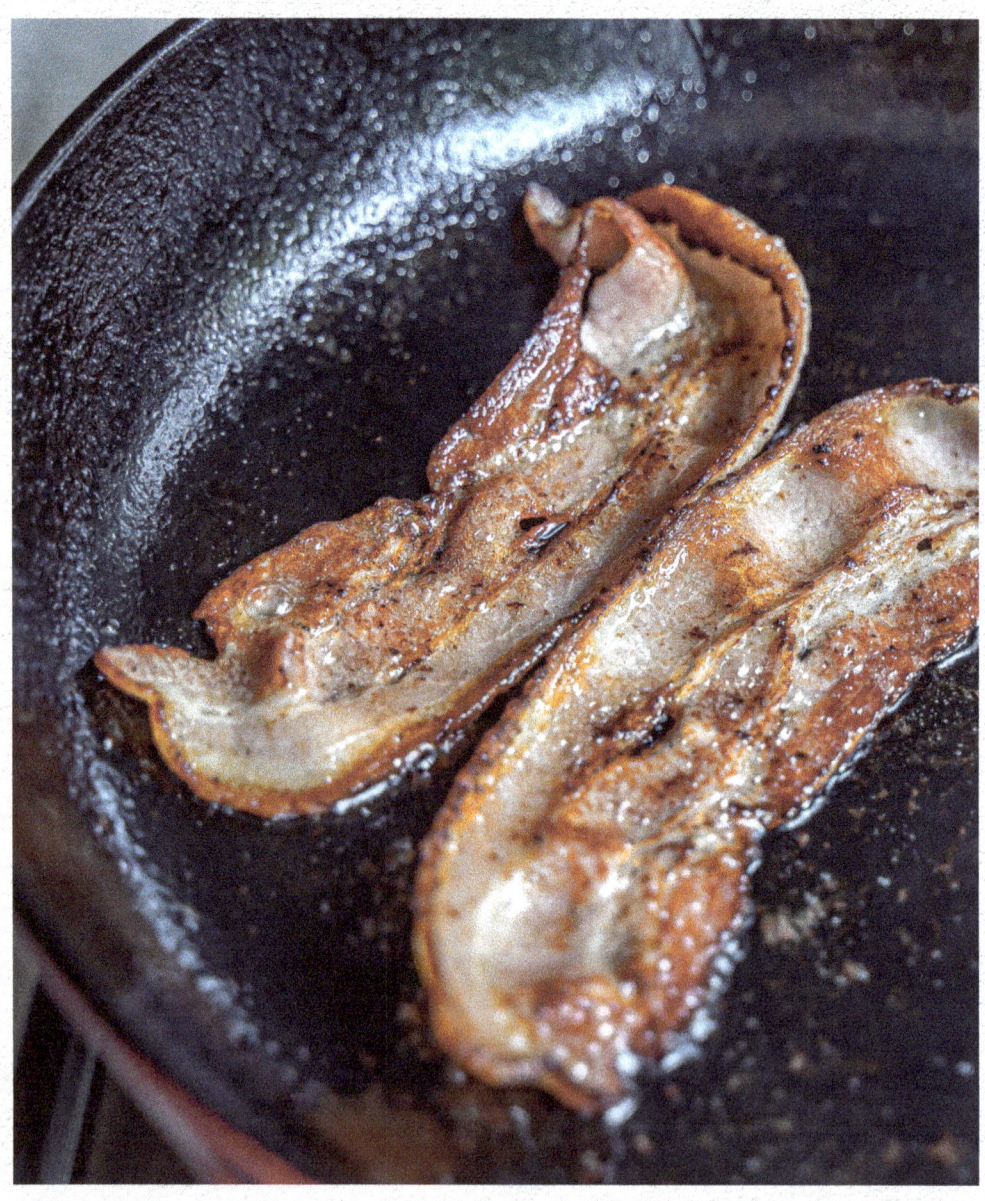

THE BURGER

2+ 100 g balls of beef mince (two or more is required to offset the sweetness)

2+ pieces of streaky bacon

2+ pieces of hi melt American cheese

Salt Flakes

2 original glazed donuts

You have two options with your bacon. Grilling is a great way to get that delicious caramelization, but you can also cook it in the oven for convenience and consistency. I like both equally; however, I find that oven cooking bacon can yield a crunchier result, which is perfect for texture. To oven bake it, place it in the oven at 180°C (356°F) for 9 minutes, then flip and cook for another 9 minutes on the other side, or until desired crunchiness. To cook it on the grill, start by preheating to a high heat and place the bacon flat on the grill and cook until the bottom has fully caramelized. Flip to the other side and cook until desired crunchiness and caramelization.

Wait until the grill is smoking hot again and place your patties on the grill one by one, leaving space between them to be flattened out.

Using your preferred smashing tool—I would suggest the best smash to do for this burger is the edged smash, purely to offset the sweetness of the donuts with a deep and crunchy caramelized edge—smash each patty to just wider than your donut. Season evenly across the patties and wait until the pink has nearly disappeared from the top. Flip your patties and place your hi melt American cheese on top of the cooked/brown side. Place your cooked bacon on top of the melting cheese. As soon as the cheese is gooey and melted, stack the patties on top of each other and remove from the grill.

Assemble your burger by placing the bacon and patties between the two donuts and applying a tablespoon of sauce just under the top donut.

Eat and enjoy!

THE MEATLOVERS PIZZA

We all have that memory of meatlovers pizza. It's a nostalgic and delicious flavor profile that has touched the heart of every young junk food lover. I distinctly remember that at the age of sixteen, after spending an afternoon attending running training with my best mate, Damo, I would order two of these pizzas just for myself. We'd spend the rest of the night with our third amigo—and other best mate—Simo, playing Battlefield Bad Company 2, knocking back about fifteen V energy drinks and eating pizza into the early hours of the morning. We'd then wake up at the lovely time of 6 a.m. and attend cycle training for another two to three hours, the night before a complete haze of video game bullets flying everywhere, excited orders shouted at each other, and memories formed forever. It's a reminder of simpler, delicious, fun times. I hope this burger brings back fond memories for you as well.

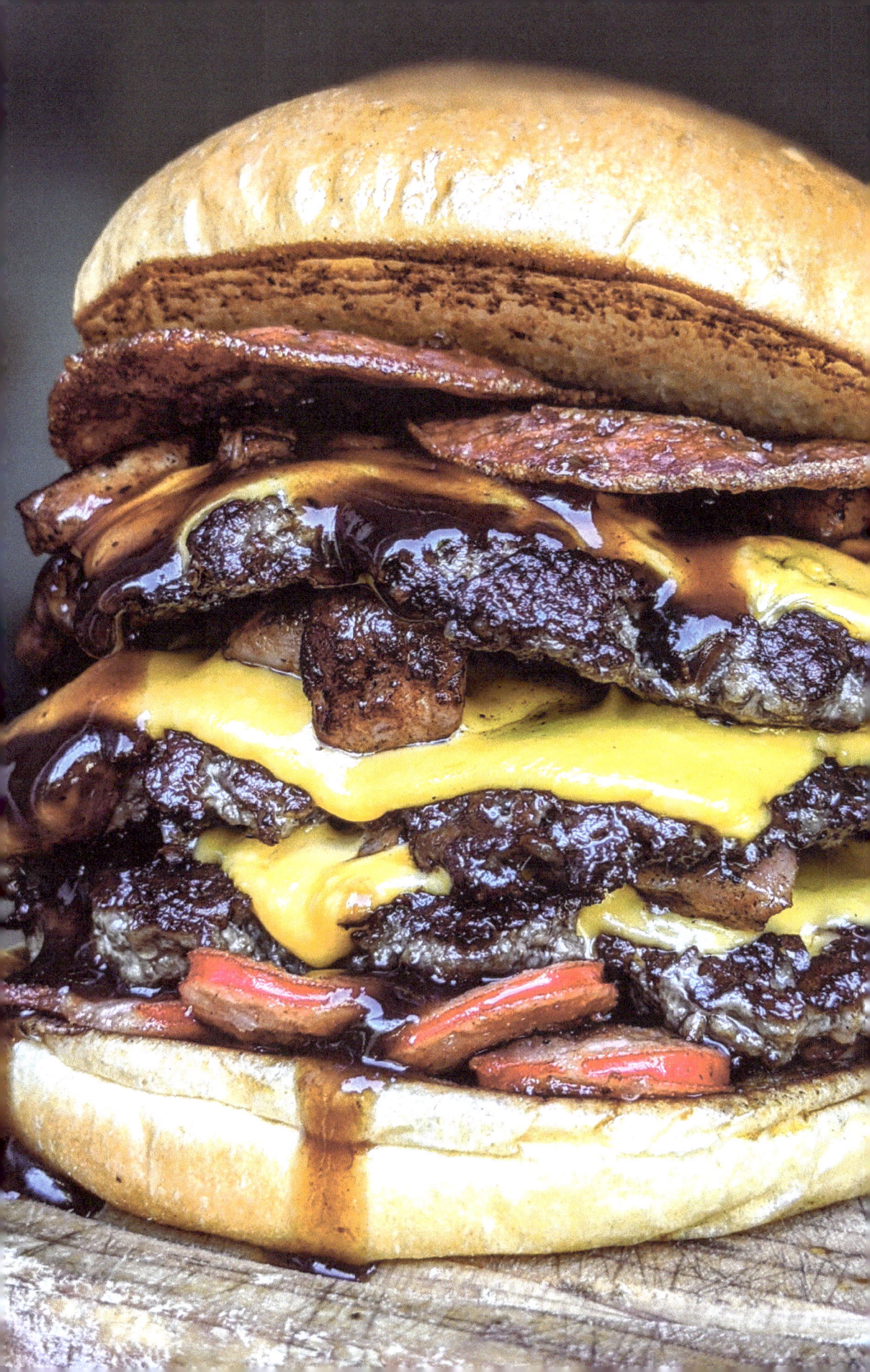

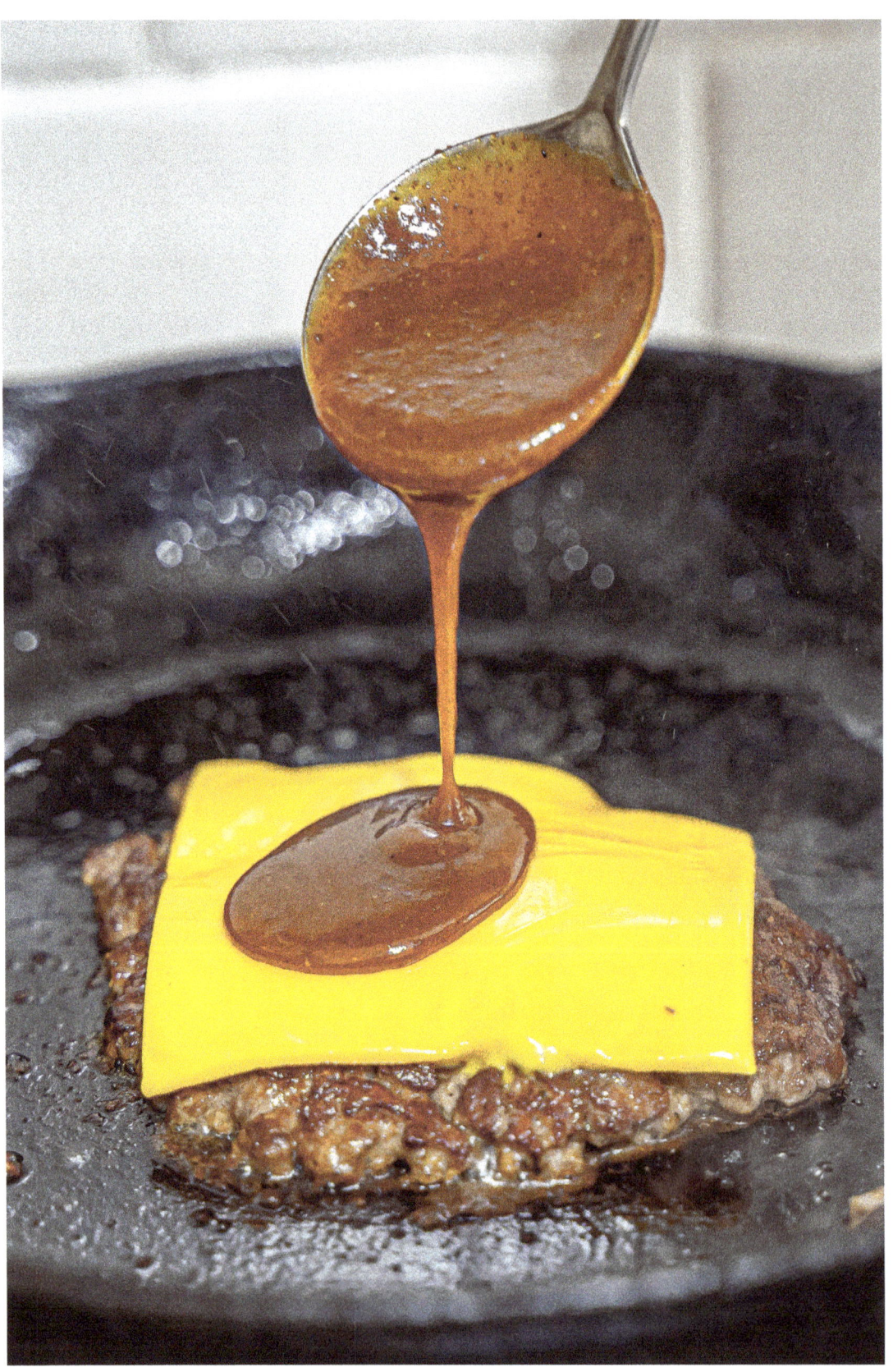

THE BURGER

2 large slices of pepperoni

1 half piece of Italian sausage

1 half stick of cabanossi

30 ml of your favorite BBQ sauce

3 x 100 g balls of beef mince

Salt flakes

1 brioche or milk bun

Start by slicing your cabanossi into 3–4 mm portions and dicing your Italian sausage into smaller uneven-sized pieces. Grill both in a cast-iron pan or on your grill until caramelized on most of the surfaces. Remove from your grill/cast-iron pan and grill both sides of the pepperoni until caramelized. Be careful with the pepperoni, as it will cook quite quickly!

Give your grill a good clean with your paint scraper and vegetable or canola oil. Heat it up to a medium heat and place the inside of your cut buns on the grill, placing a small amount of pressure on them. Wait until they become soft and airy, and slightly brown on the inside. Remove and put aside for later.

Put the grill on high and wait until it is smoking hot. Place your patties on the grill one by one, leaving space between them to be flattened out.

Using your preferred smashing tool—you can either opt for a flat smash or an edged smash—press down your patties to just wider than your bun width. Season evenly across the patties and wait until the pink has nearly disappeared from the top. Flip your patties and place your hi melt American cheese on top of the cooked/brown side. Place the cooked Italian sausage on two of the patties and put the cooked pepperoni on the patty you intend to have on the top layer. As soon as the cheese is melted, stack the patties on top of each other, with the pepperoni patty on top, and remove from the grill.

Assemble your burger by placing the cooked cabanossi on top of the bottom bun, stacking your patties on top, and saucing your burger to preferred sauciness with your favorite BBQ sauce.

Eat and enjoy!

THE MI GORENG

I don't know about you, but I feel like everyone I know has their own mi goreng story: whether it was their backpacking trip across Europe, where they needed a cheap and easy option to take everywhere, or the classic dorm room snack for those down on cash that week. For me, it has had many appearances in different parts of my life. It started with a year ten camp, where we stayed in a hostel and were budgeted $5 a day for food. It appeared again when I was a fresh-faced eighteen year old, moved out of home, earning $12.50 an hour, with a couple of parking fines that almost bankrupted me. Finally, I had the classic uni student experience, eating it in between classes, trying to fill a rumbling belly while I studied—or at least pretended to. Mi goreng is another nostalgic flavor that keeps coming back for more, and it's a true classic. Here's just one way you can add those flavors to your burger.

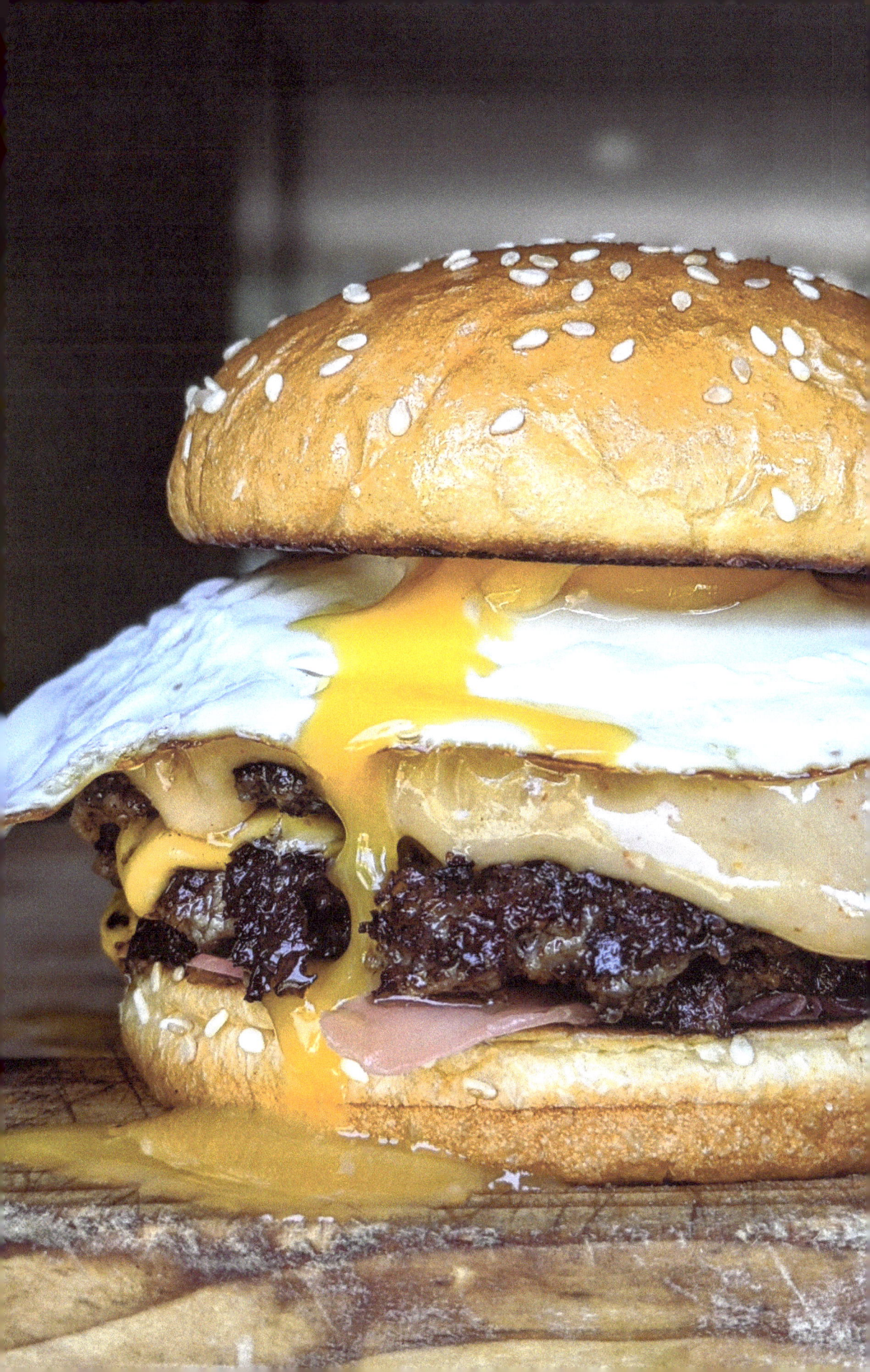

THE SAUCE

60 g of whole egg mayonnaise

1 packet of mi goreng

In a small mixing bowl, empty out all the ingredients from the mi goreng flavor packets. Add the whole egg mayonnaise and mix together until it's a smooth and consistent texture.

THE BURGER

1–3 x 120 g balls of beef mince

1–3 slices of American hi melt cheese

1 extra-large egg

30 g of pickled ginger

Salt flakes

10 ml of canola oil

1 brioche or milk bun

20 g of fried shallots (not included in video)

Preheat a nonstick pan to a low-medium heat. Add the oil into the pan and coat evenly. Crack your egg, pour it onto the heated nonstick pan, and cook on a low temp until all the white is cooked but the yolk is still runny.

Give your grill a good clean with your paint scraper and vegetable or canola oil. Heat it up to a medium heat and place the inside of your cut buns on the grill, placing a small amount of pressure on them. Wait until they become soft and airy, and slightly brown on the inside. Remove and put aside for later.

Cut your bun in half.

Put the grill on high and wait until it is smoking hot. Place your patties on the grill one by one, leaving space between them to be flattened out.

Using your preferred smashing tool—you can either opt for a flat smash or an edged smash—press down your patties to just wider than your bun width. Season evenly across the patties and wait until the pink has nearly disappeared from the top. Flip your patties and place your hi melt American cheese on top of the cooked/brown side.

Assemble your burger by placing the pickled ginger on the bottom bun, the patties on top, then the egg, some fried shallots, and finish with your top bun and mi goreng sauce.

Eat and enjoy!

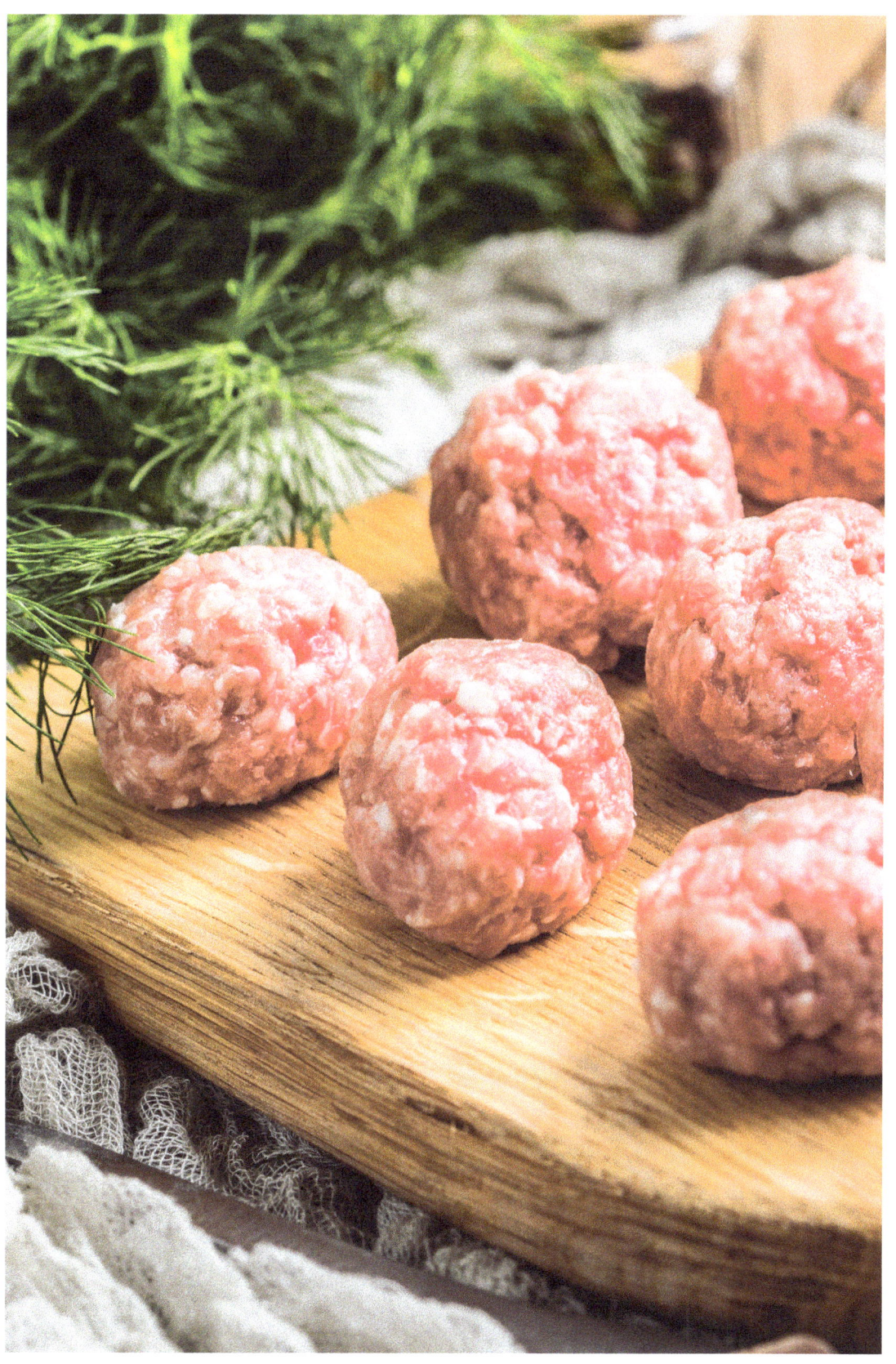

THE FAT FRYDAY

Every good cheat meal recipe book needs something—if not everything—fried. Cheese is possibly the easiest go-to for food porn and cheat meals, and adding Doritos just gives it a whole other stoner vibe. I love a good fried cheese. It adds texture to a burger with that delicious crunchy exterior and oozing comforting cheesy goodness on the inside. The most important thing when frying cheese is to make sure that it's *completely* coated before deep frying; otherwise, it leaks, and you lose half of your cheese. To be completely honest, for this recipe, the burger is almost identical to the OG, so it's nothing groundbreaking. I wanted the Dorito fried cheese to be the hero of the burger, so, really, you can add it to any other simple burger recipe in this book for extra calories and yumminess.

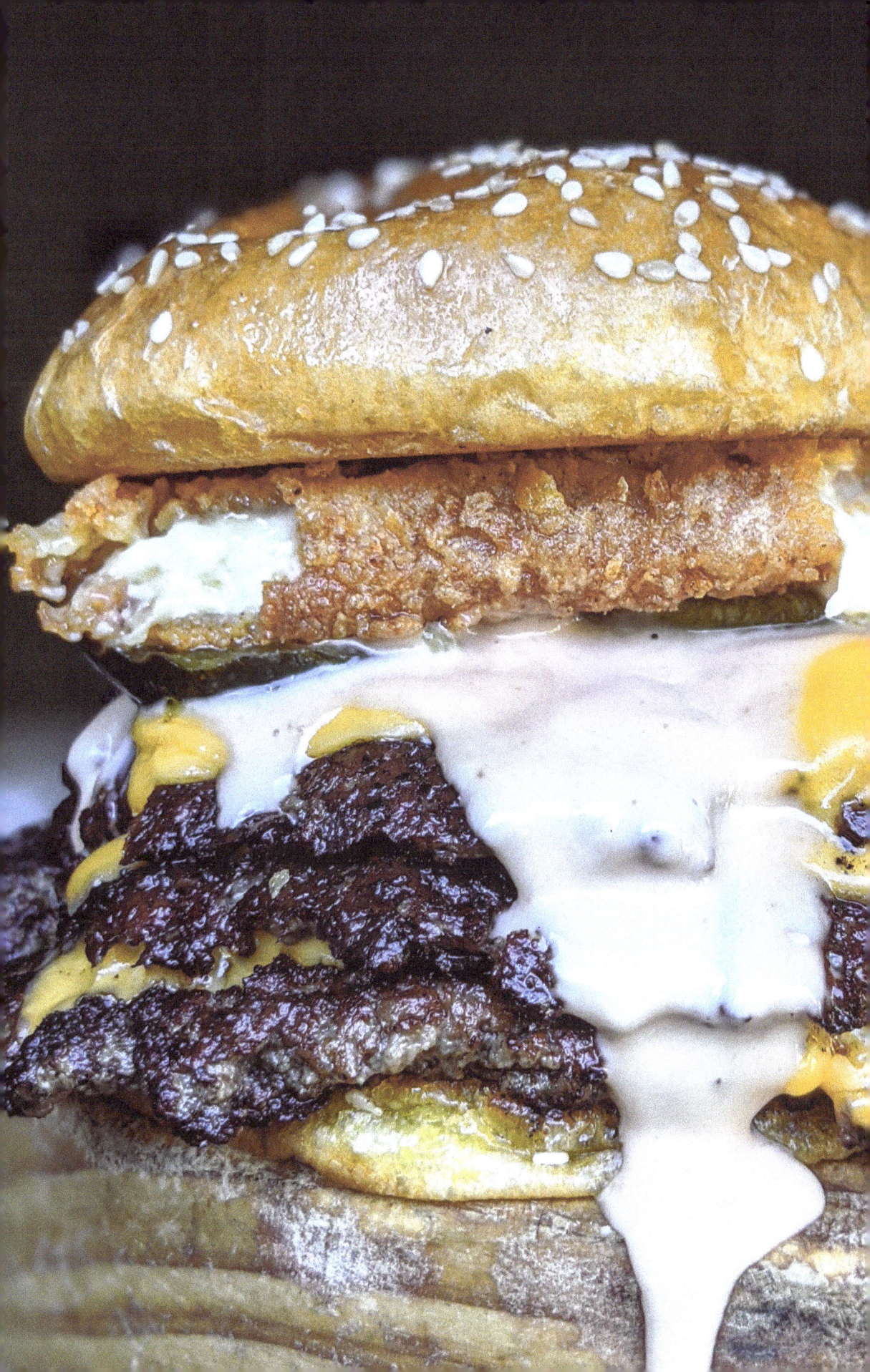

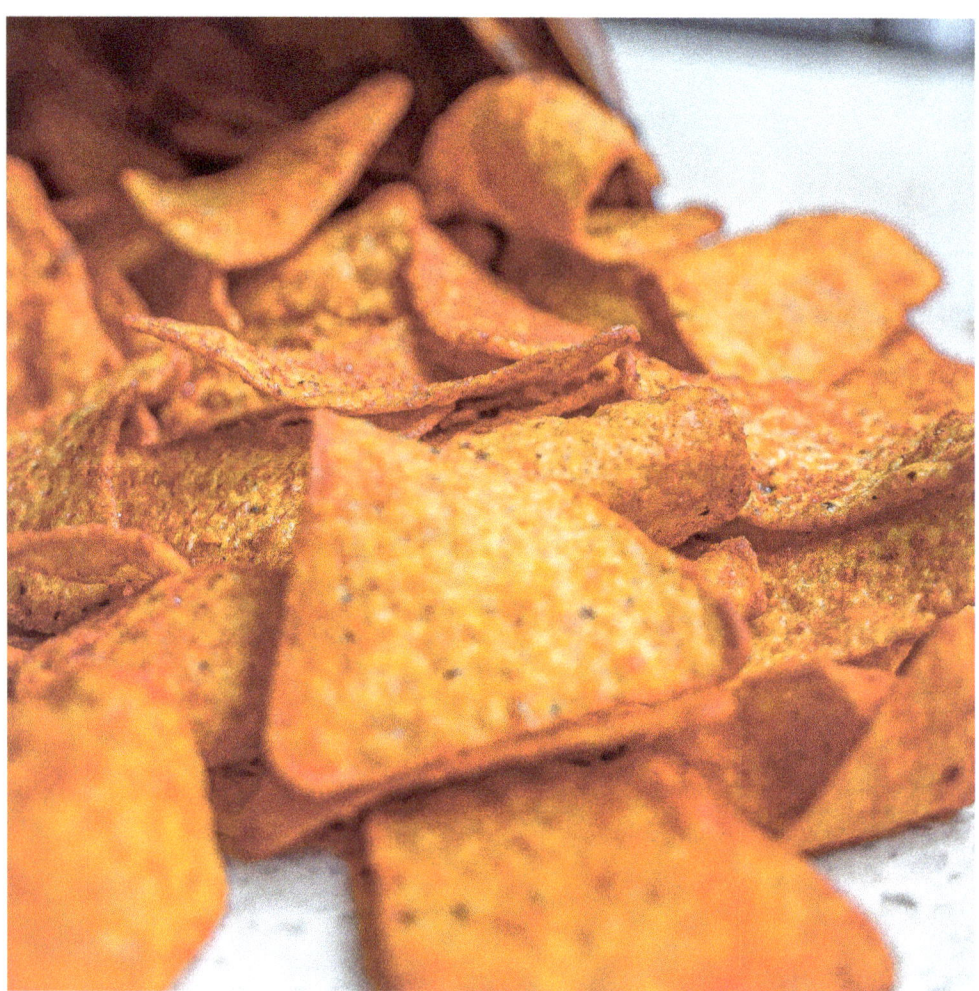

THE FRIED CHEESE

1 cup of crushed Doritos

½ cup of plain flour

½ cup of corn flour

1 tsp of smoked paprika

1 tsp of onion powder

1 tsp of garlic powder

1 tsp of ground white pepper

1 large slice of mozzarella or provolone, 7–8 mm thick

2 x large eggs

3 L of canola oil

Mix all the dry ingredients for the fried cheese in a large mixing bowl and whisk together to break up any bits of flour and spices.

Crack your two eggs into a small mixing bowl and whisk until the egg wash is consistent in color and all mixed in.

Place the cheese in the egg mix until completely covered, then place it in the Dorito flour mix and coat evenly. Remove from the flour and give a light shake to remove any loose bits.

Preheat your grill to high temperature prior to cooking your fried cheese.

THE SAUCE

60 g of whole egg mayonnaise
40 g of ketchup
20 ml of sweet pickle juice

Create your sauce. Put all the ingredients together and mix with a spoon until smooth and creamy. This part of the recipe is discretional, and you can interchange the ingredients at different ratios to your preference. Once mixed, store in the fridge.

THE BURGER

1–3 x 120 g balls of beef mince
1–3 slices of American hi melt cheese
Sweet pickles
Soft milk or brioche bun
Salt flakes

Prepare your beef into equally sized balls, using either store-bought, butcher's, or homemade mince. Place in the fridge uncovered for 10 minutes prior to cooking

Cut your milk or brioche bun in half.

Heat your oil or deep fryer to 170°C (338°F). Place the flour-coated cheese in and cook until the exterior is crisp and brown. Once removed, allow it to cool down while you cook your burger.

Place the inside of your cut buns on the grill, placing a small amount of pressure on them. Wait until they become soft and airy, and slightly brown on the inside. Remove and put aside for assembly.

Wait until the grill is smoking hot and place your patties on the grill one by one, leaving space between them to be flattened out.

Using your preferred smashing tool—you can either opt for a flat smash or an edged smash—press down your patties to just wider than your bun width. Season evenly across the patties and wait until the pink has nearly disappeared from the top. Flip your patties and place your hi melt American cheese on top of the cooked/brown side. As soon as the cheese is melted, you can remove the patties from the grill and prepare to assemble your burger.

Assemble your burger by repeating the steps in the **OG burger recipe**, and then place the fried cheese on top of the patties. Eat and enjoy!

THE HOLY GUACAMOLE

Hands down, if you were to take burgers and barbecue out this world, as much as that would be sad, Mexican cuisine would be my next favorite food to eat. I love spice. I grew up in an interesting household, where an Indian curry was as much a staple as a good spaghetti Bolognese in most families. My dad and the previous three generations of my family lived in the beautiful country of Fiji. They brought such amazing cultural richness back to Australia, whether it was the carefree "Fiji time" attitude, great sense of humor, or incredible ability to be inclusive of everyone. They also brought the delicious Indian cuisine back with them because nearly half of Fiji is inhabited by Indians.

So, I grew up with my Narni (grandmother) cooking us all sorts of delectable and spiced-up curries. It was amazing. I grew up with an intense love for spiced food, which has always made me favor Mexican. Lucky enough for me, the beautiful Mrs. Food Coma (Kira) also loves it, and she coerced me into making the both of us a burger featuring some elements found in Mexican food. This turned out to be one of my favorite recipes and really grew my love for fusing different cuisines into my burgers.

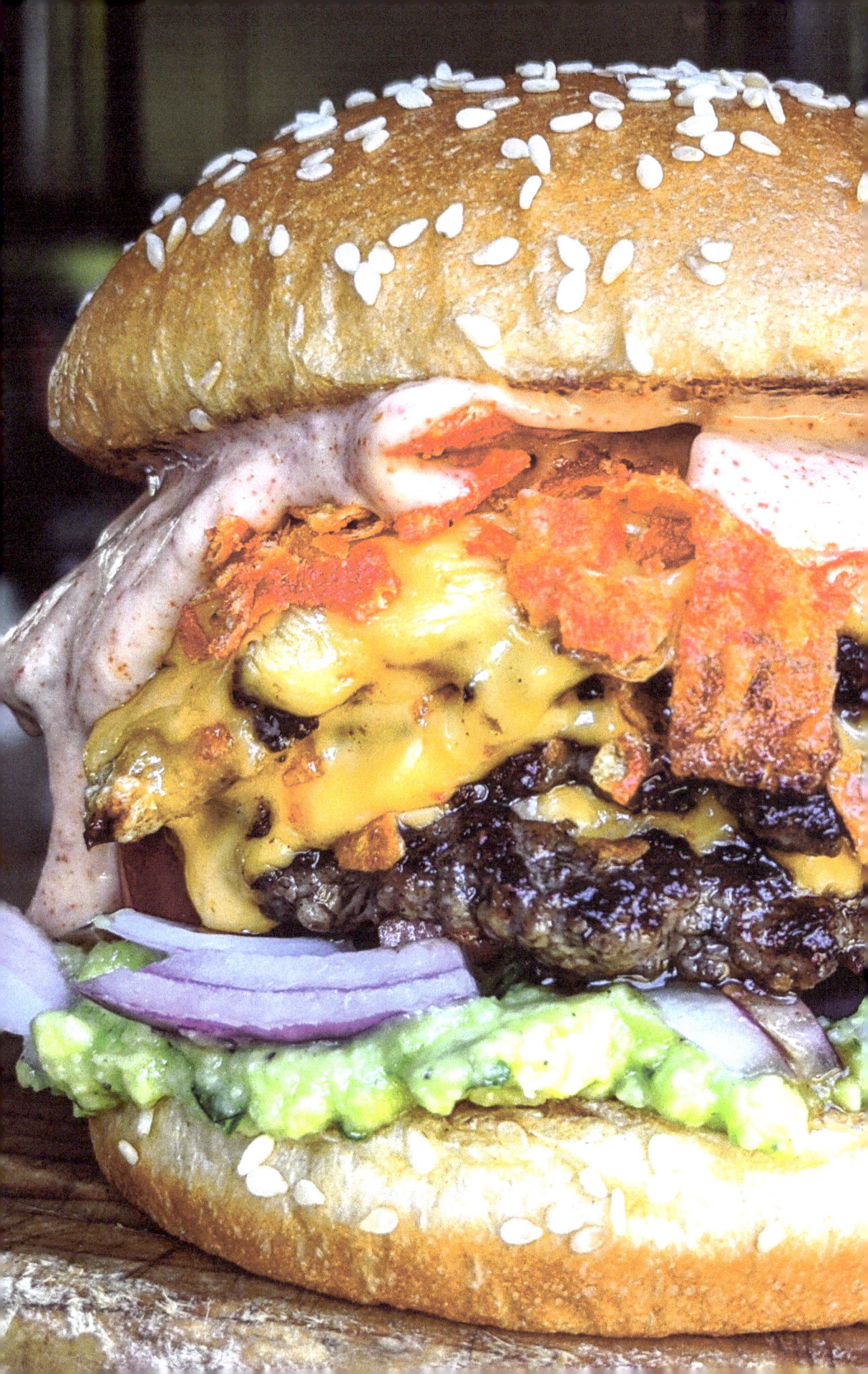

THE SAUCE

30 ml Byron Bay Chilli Co. mango and habanero hot sauce (or a similar alternative)

60 ml whole egg mayonnaise

1 pinch of smoked paprika

20 ml of lemon juice

Create your sauce. Put all the ingredients together and mix with a spoon until smooth and creamy. This part of the recipe is discretional, and you can interchange the ingredients at different ratios to your preference. Once mixed, store it in the fridge.

THE GUACAMOLE

½ avocado

Salt

Pepper

Fresh coriander (not mandatory, but I love it)

30 ml of lemon juice

Prepare your guacamole by slicing your avocado in half, removing the pit, and emptying the contents into a small mixing bowl. Finely slice your coriander into small flakes. Add salt, pepper (depending on how strong you like it) and your sliced coriander. Mush the contents together with a fork until it's a chunky consistency. Add a squeeze of lemon and mix again. It should be quite chunky but mixed evenly.

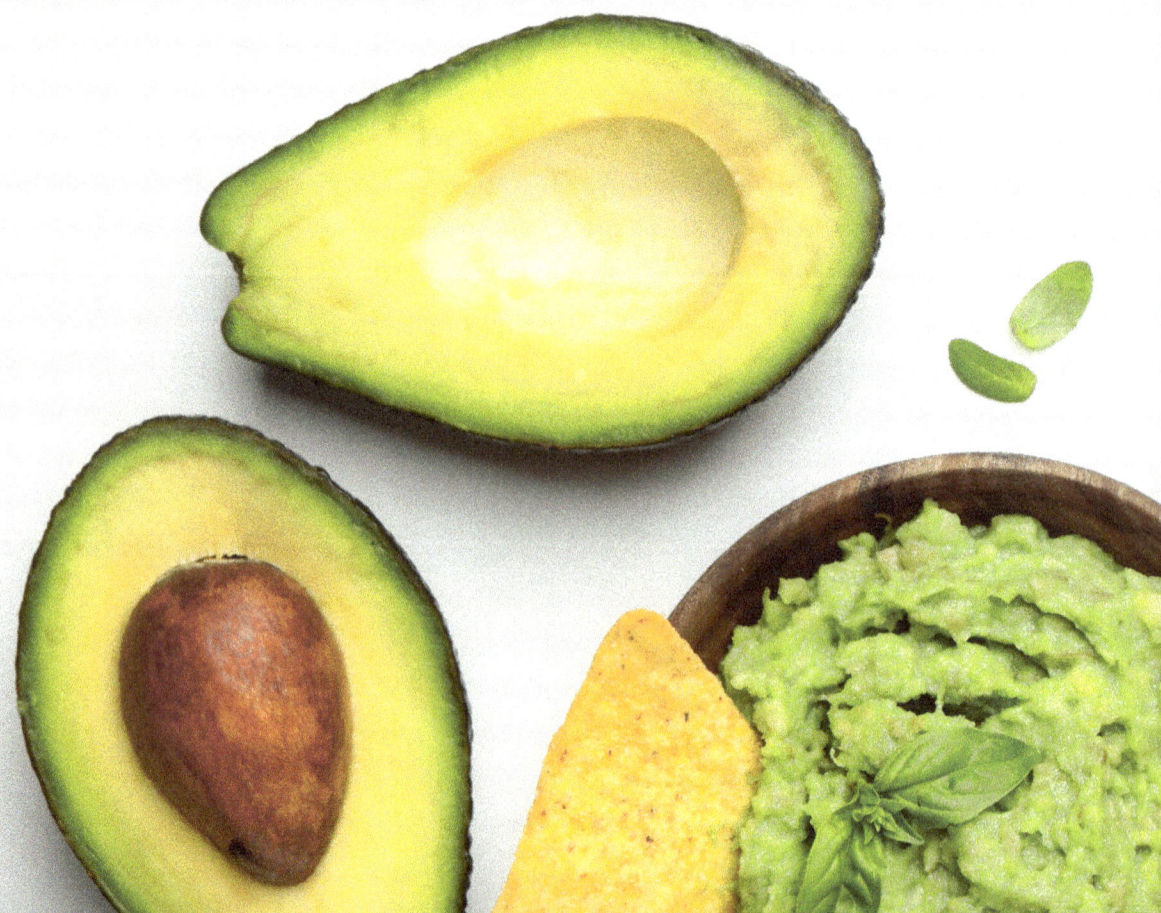

THE BURGER

Half a handful of crushed Doritos corn chips

1–3 x 100 g balls of beef mince

1–3 slices of American hi melt cheese

Salt flakes

1 brioche or milk bun

¼ of a tomato

¼ of a red onion

Dice your tomato and red onion into equally sized pieces, cutting approximately 20–30 g of each.

Slice your bun in half.

Preheat your grill to a medium heat.

Place the inside of your cut buns on the grill, placing a small amount of pressure on them. Wait until they become soft and airy, and slightly brown on the inside. Remove and put aside for assembly.

Heat your grill up to a high temperature, wait until it's smoking hot, and place your patties on the grill one by one, leaving space between them to be flattened out.

Using your preferred smashing tool—you can either opt for a flat smash or an edged smash—press down your patties to just wider than your bun width. Season evenly across the patties and wait until the pink has nearly disappeared from the top. Flip your patties and place your hi melt American cheese on top of the cooked/brown side. Add your crushed corn chips to each patty and as soon as the cheese is melted, you can remove the patties from the grill and prepare to assemble your burger.

Assemble your burger in the following order: bottom bun, guacamole, red onion, tomato, patties, sauce, and finally, top bun.

Eat and enjoy!

THE BACON ME CRAZY

My favorite ever condiment to put on a burger—other than the burger patty itself—is hands down, unequivocally, a delicious, mouthwatering, sweet, smoky, spicy and savory bacon jam. It truly is a special ingredient that adds so many different elements to a burger's flavor and texture profile. My Instagram has been flooded with messages asking what my bacon jam recipe is, and the chaotic part is that I make it different every time. I like to free-pour ingredients and if they're in general ratios, it always tastes delicious. I've livestreamed making it; I've made about seven different videos featuring it, and each time I have not weighed out a single ingredient. That must drive some people mental, but I like the freeness of it. I will try my best to put this recipe down in exact terms for you so that you can experience it close to how I envisage it. I spent so long writing about bacon jam that I forgot to mention the other ingredients! But really, the bacon jam is the hero; the rest of the ingredients are just reminiscent of what a twelve-week dieter's sweat-induced dream would look like.

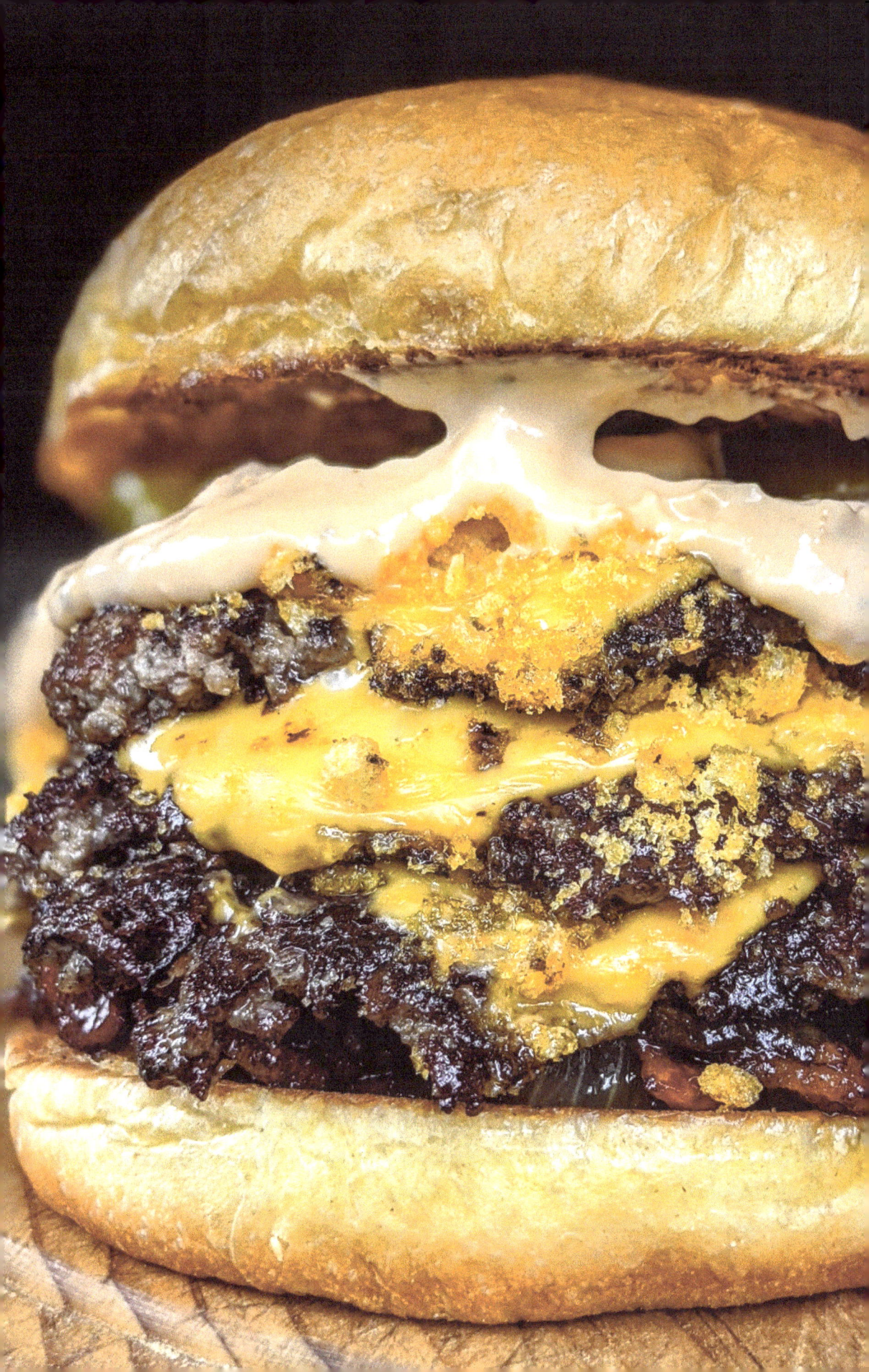

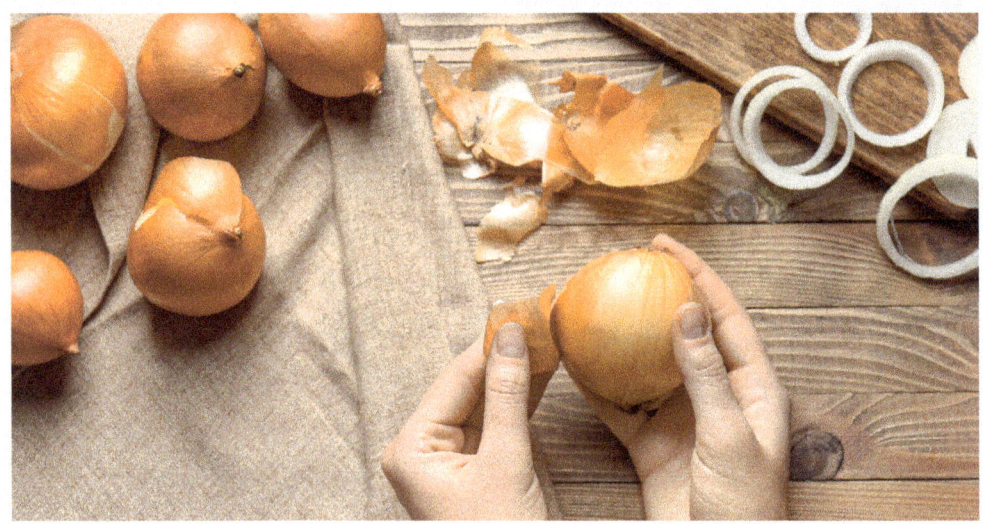

BACON JAM

1 large onion

2–3 French shallots

½ cup of maple syrup

⅛ cup of Maker's Mark Bourbon (not included in the video)

½ cup of brown sugar

¼ cup of apple cider vinegar

1 tsp of cayenne pepper powder

½ kg of streaky bacon

3 cloves of garlic

Finely dice your large onion and shallots. You can either mince the garlic or crush with the flat part of a knife and finely dice. Alternatively, you can cheat by using an already-minced garlic product from your local supermarket.

Cut your bacon into equal-size squares, approximately 2 cm in width/height.

Start by cooking down your bacon in a large nonstick pot until it's fully caramelized and a deep red/brown. Remove from the pot through a strainer and place the leftover bacon fat back into the pot.

Throw your onion, garlic, and shallots in the pot with the leftover bacon fat. Leave on a medium heat and stir every 1 minute with a wooden spoon until they're browned.

Once the onion, garlic and shallots are cooked, place the cooked bacon back into the pot and stir together until mixed in. Put the rest of your ingredients in and stir slowly on a medium heat. Once everything is mixed in, cook on a low heat and reduce the liquid until you have a thick mixture, with slowly rising, almost lazy-looking, bubbles. Remove from heat and place aside for burger assembly.

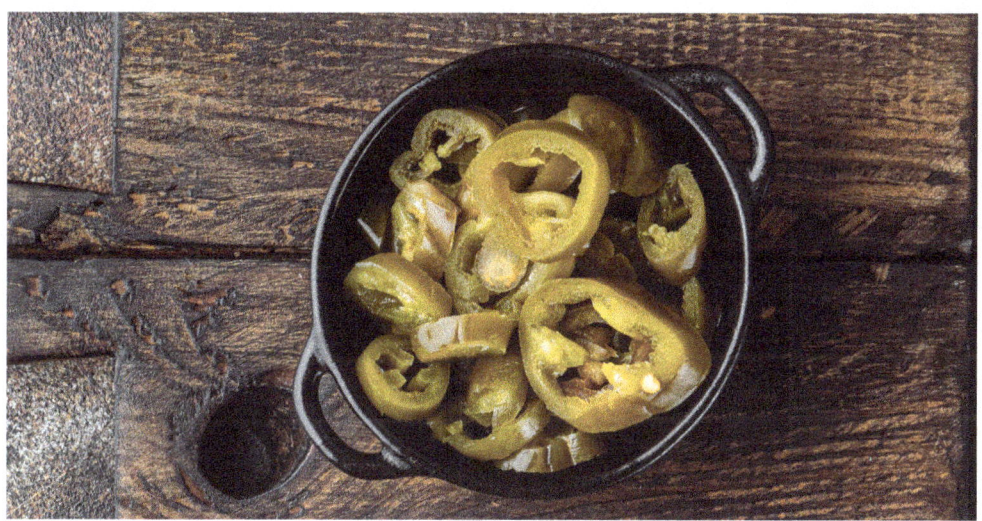

THE BURGER

- ¼ cup of crushed Twisties
- 1–3 100 g balls of beef mince
- 30 ml of Heinz baconnaise (or a similar alternative)
- 1–3 slices of American hi melt cheese
- 4 slices of pickled jalapeños
- 1 brioche or milk bun

Crush your Twisties in either a sealed ziplock back using a rolling pin or with a mortar and pestle.

Slice your brioche/milk bun in half.

Preheat your grill to a medium heat.

Place the inside of your cut buns on the grill, placing a small amount of pressure on them. Wait until they become soft and airy, and slightly brown on the inside. Remove and put aside for assembly.

Heat your grill up to a high temperature, wait until it is smoking hot, and place your patties on the grill one by one, leaving space between them to be flattened out.

Using your preferred smashing tool—you can either opt for a flat smash or an edged smash—press down your patties to just wider than your bun width. Season evenly across the patties and wait until the pink has nearly disappeared from the top. Flip your patties and place your hi melt American cheese on top of the cooked/brown side. Add your crushed Twisties to each patty and as soon as the cheese is melted, you can remove the patties from the grill and prepare to assemble your burger.

Assemble your burger. Eat and enjoy!

THE OKTOBERFEST

Oktoberfest only comes around once a year, but, in reality, I wish it could be every couple of months. First of all, beer is bloody delicious. I thoroughly enjoy a cold one straight from the tap. That first sip is almost like nirvana: a crisp hoppy freshness hits your tongue and swishes around your mouth, bringing with it an effervescence, making you feel just that little bit more alive. I forgot for a second that I was supposed to be talking about burgers.

With good beer, comes good old-fashioned German food: schnitzels, sauerkraut, pork knuckles, bratwursts, and so much more. I have been known to smash a stein of Hofbräu, knock back 1 kg of veal or chicken schnitzel, and celebrate the feast with delicious, flavored schnapps. I wanted to bring forward those amazingly moreish flavors in a burger, and this is what I came up with. Bear in mind, the sausage in this recipe is completely interchangeable with whatever German sausage takes your fancy. The most important thing is that you enjoy it.

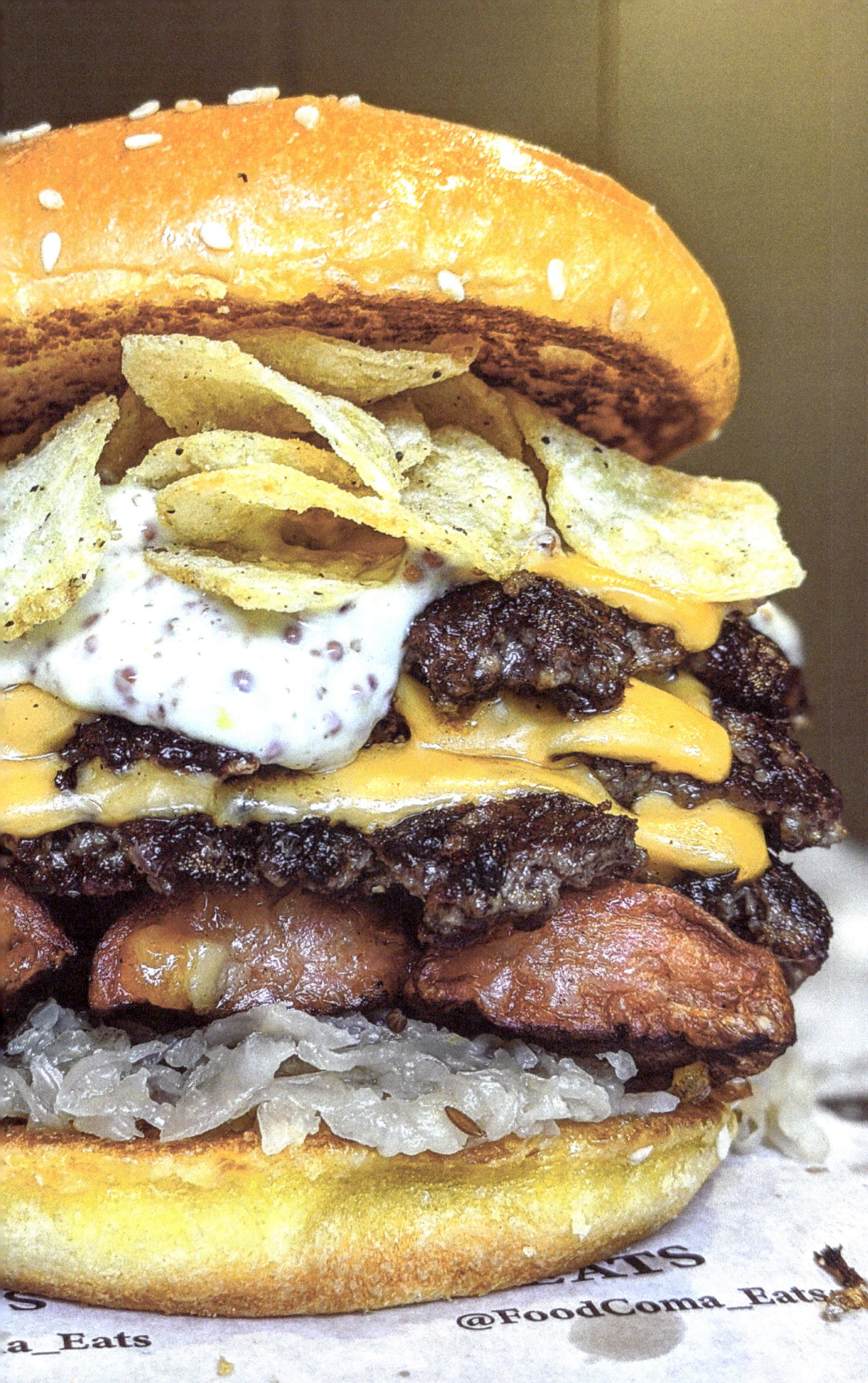

THE SAUCE

60 ml of whole egg mayonnaise

30 ml of whole grain mustard

Prepare your sauce by mixing the ingredients together until grainy and consistent in texture. Put aside for assembly.

THE BURGER

¾ of a knackwurst sausage (smoked German sausage)

30–40 g of jarred sauerkraut

Handful of salt-flavored crisps

1 brioche or milk bun

1–3 100 g balls of beef mince

1–3 slices of American hi melt cheese (can be swapped for a nutty Jarlsberg cheese)

Slice your knackwurst sausage in half, then split it lengthways to make 4 equal portions.

Grill all 4 quarter-sized pieces in a cast-iron pan or grill at a medium heat until browned on the outside. Reward yourself for all your hard work by eating one of the said sausage quarters.

Slice your brioche/milk bun in half.

Preheat your grill to a medium heat.

Place the inside of your cut buns on the grill, placing a small amount of pressure on them. Wait until they become soft and airy, and slightly brown on the inside. Remove and put aside for assembly.

Heat your grill up to a high temperature, wait until it's smoking hot, and place your patties on the grill one by one, leaving space between them to be flattened out.

Using your preferred smashing tool—you can either opt for a flat smash or an edged smash—press down your patties to just wider than your bun width. Season evenly across the patties and wait until the pink has nearly disappeared from the top. Flip your patties and place your hi melt American cheese on top of the cooked/brown side. As soon as the cheese is melted, you can remove the patties from the grill and prepare to assemble your burger.

Assemble all ingredients onto your burger. Eat and enjoy!

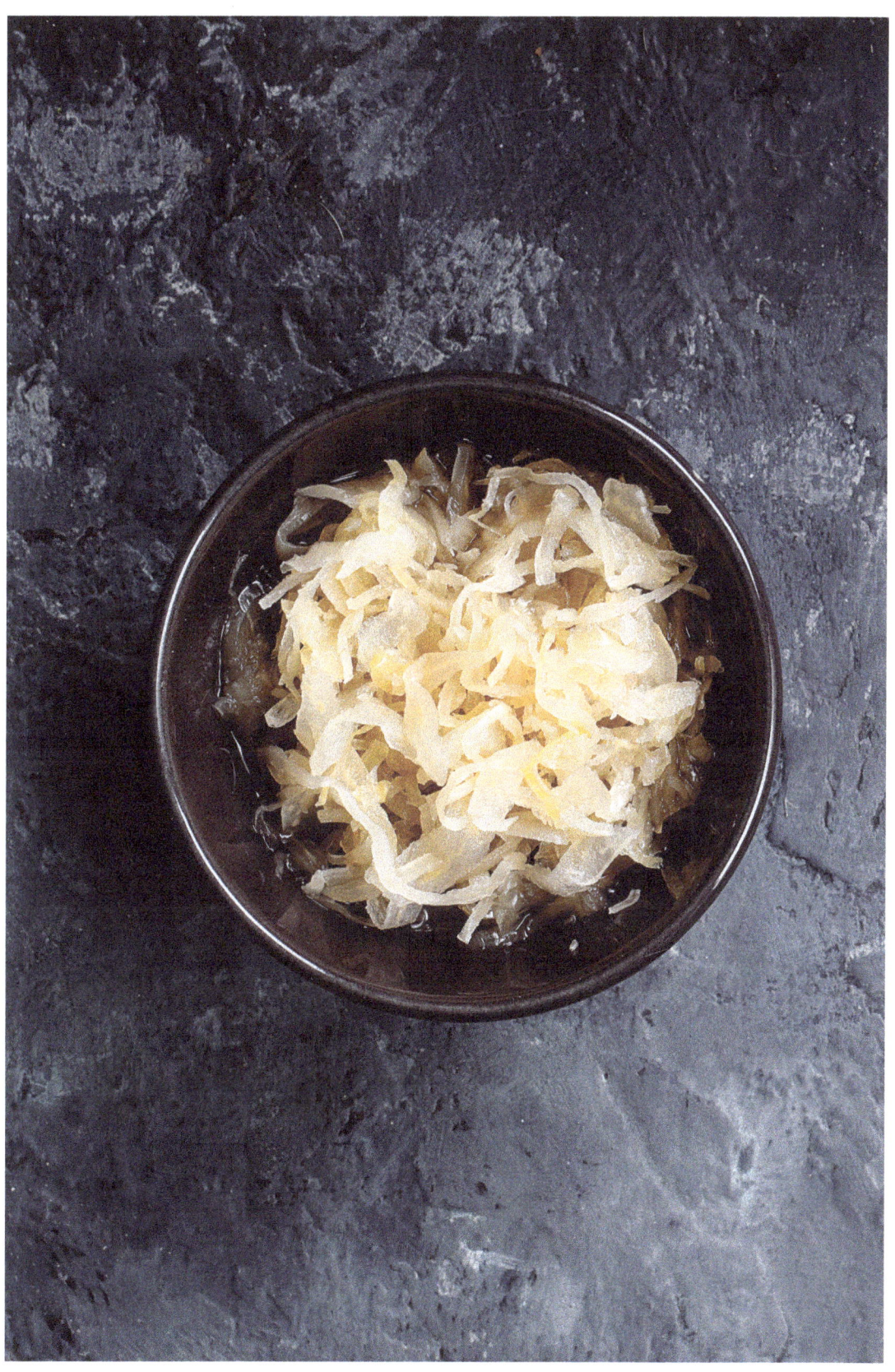

THE SIMPLE SANDO

Shock and horror—there's something included in this book that's not technically a burger! In fact, there's going to be a few recipes in this book that are not strictly burgers, so shut your yapper, get some sandwiches in your gob, and move on, because I don't discriminate. In all seriousness, there are blurred lines across the industry on what constitutes a burger, and what is a sandwich. I've always held that if something does not include ground beef, it cannot be a burger. But that hasn't ever stopped me from creating sandwiches that are built much like burgers. The key difference is the protein that goes into it.

In this case, it's a simple fried chicken sandwich. If you do a Google search, I almost promise you that you will be able to find 1,700 different fried chicken recipes. It's a staple cheat meal food and one of my favorite things to eat. My recipe is no better than anyone else's; it's just what I like and how I like to do it. That being said, I have learned a few interesting tricks and tips along the way to make sure you get a solid product every single time.

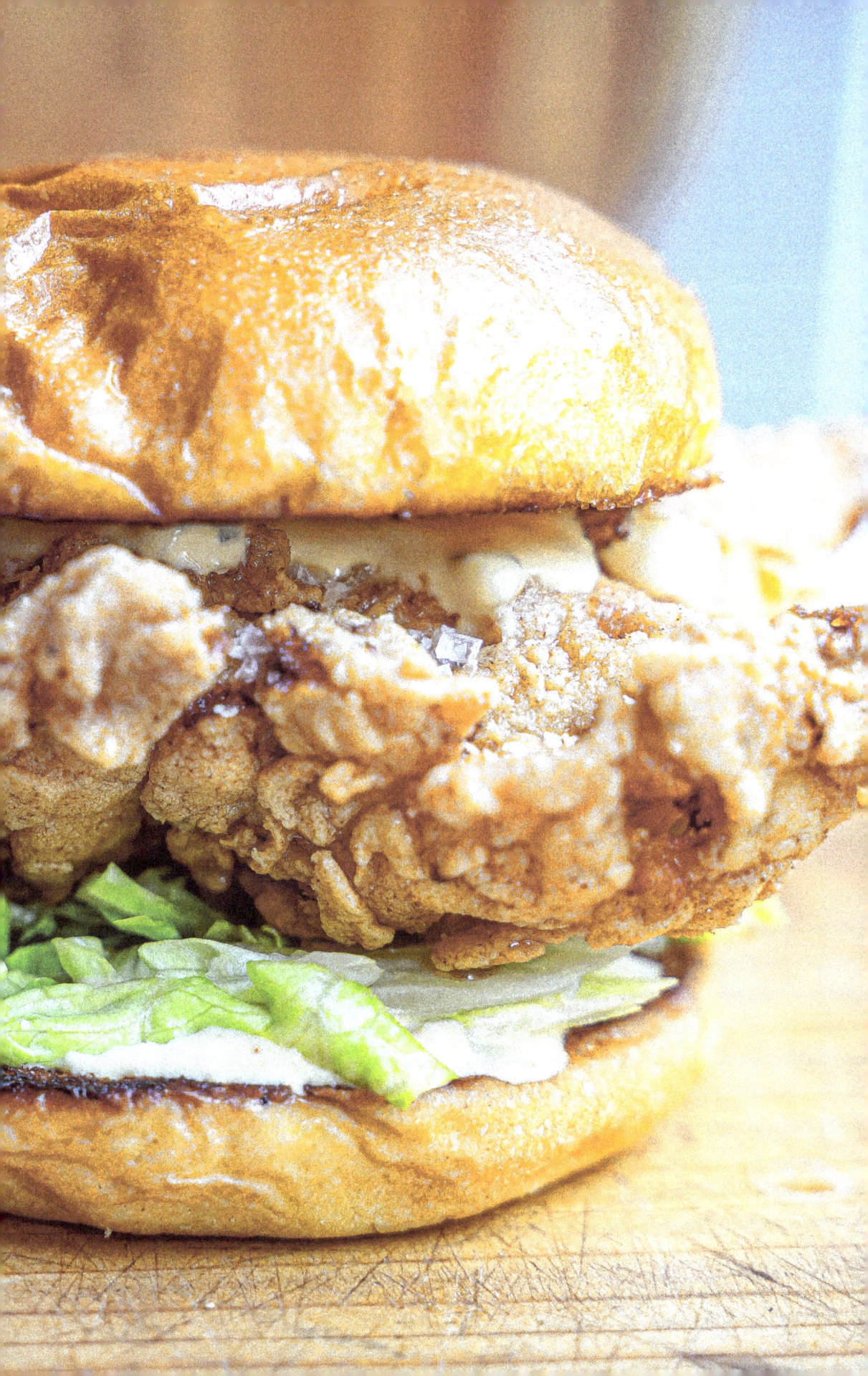

FOOD COMA FRIED CHICKEN HOT TIPS

- Save yourself some hassle and wear gloves when flouring your chicken. Once you're done, instead of spending 3–5 minutes cleaning the sticky batter off your hands, you can just remove the gloves and place them in the bin.

- The bigger the bowl for your seasoned flour, the better. There will be more room for you to work with, and it's a lot easier to cover the chicken fully in flour.

- Play around with your flour ratios and even which starches you use in the process. You get a completely different product when you use things like chickpea flour, rice flour, potato flour, corn starch, and plain flour.

- Don't fixate on your flour being perfectly smooth. Little bits of clumpy flour can add a delicious texture to your fried chicken.

FOR THE FRYER

- Get your hands on a dedicated deep fryer. They can be as cheap as $20 AUD and will help you control the temp of the oil a lot easier than a pot.

- Make sure you replace your oil once it starts to get dark and dirty from too many cooks.

- Your oil heat is incredibly important and will depend on the size of your product. Larger/thicker fillets and tenders may be better cooked at 170°C (338°F) oil heat. Thinner products may need a higher heat of around 180°C (356°F). You want the inside of your chicken to be cooked through, with a nice, crispy exterior that's not overcooked.

FOR THE CHICKEN

- For a juicier result, brine your chicken for 6–12 hours prior to cooking.

- Season your chicken like you would a burger. Either using salt or a custom spice mix, lightly dust your fillets or tenders evenly after you have finished deep frying them.

- Start with a product that's as dry as possible. Pat down each fillet or tender prior to placing in buttermilk and frying; this will help the batter adhere to the chicken better.

- If you don't have time to brine, start by flouring your chicken in plain flour first, then dip in buttermilk, and finish with your seasoned flour. This will help keep the chicken from losing its batter.

- Double flouring your chicken—which is when you flour normally and then place the chicken back in the buttermilk and seasoned flour again for a thicker layer—can make for a great crunchy fillet. But sometimes it can mean that you get an unappealing batter/chicken ratio. If you are hell-bent on double flouring, try using a thinner wet product when you transition between the layers of seasoned flour. Milk works great; I've also heard of people using salted water before—seriously it works—or you can always opt for the trusty egg.

- Always shake the loose bits off your chicken once you are done drenching it in flour. The more loose bits, the higher the chance of your batter falling off.

THE CHICKEN

200 ml of buttermilk

150–180 g fillet of chicken thigh

Place your chicken thigh into a bowl of buttermilk and leave covered for 6–12 hours to brine in the fridge.

THE FLOUR

½ cup of plain flour

½ cup of corn flour

1 tsp of smoked paprika

1 tsp of onion powder

1 tsp of garlic powder

1 tsp of ground white pepper

1 tsp of cayenne pepper

1 tsp of chipotle powder (if you can find it, not mandatory)

Prepare your seasoned flour by placing all the ingredients together in a large mixing bowl and whisking together until fully mixed.

Heat your deep fryer to 170°C (338°F).

Remove your chicken from the fridge and pull it out of the buttermilk, giving it a shake to stop any dripping. Place the fillet in the seasoned flour and cover it completely with the mixture. Put a small amount of pressure on the covered fillet, then flip it over and repeat by covering in flour again. Once again, place a small amount of pressure on the fillet, then remove from the flour and give it a light shake to remove any loose bits. Repeat for as many fillets as you intend to cook.

Place the fillet in the deep fryer basket and submerge in the oil, giving it a little shake to stop the fillet from sticking to the metal. If you intend to put the fillet straight into the oil, **be careful of splash back**. Oil burns are the worst.

Cook the chicken until golden brown on the outside, approximately 10–12 minutes. Do not rush this process. Nobody wants to get salmonella. If you have a particularly thick piece of chicken, consider slicing it in half at the thickest part and checking to see whether it has any raw bits.

Turn over to the next page to continue with the recipe

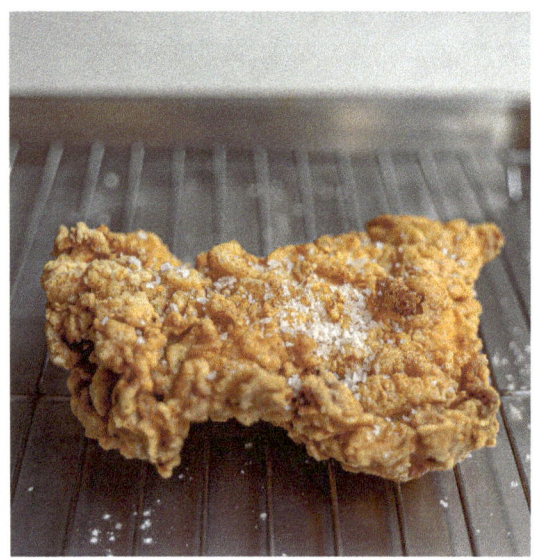
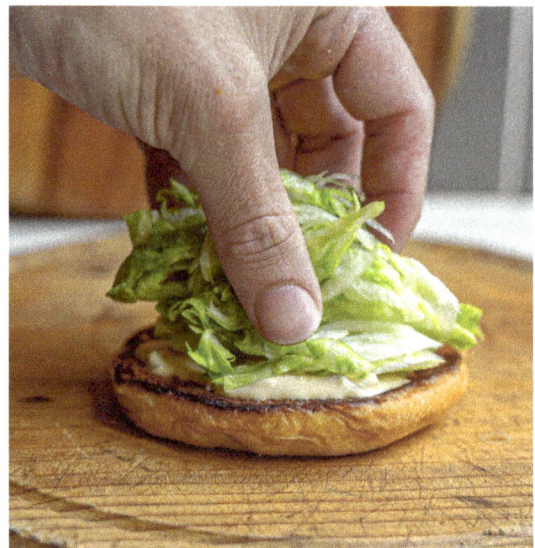

THE BURGER

60 g of shredded iceberg lettuce

1 brioche or milk bun

While your chicken is cooking, quickly slice your iceberg into thin and crunchy pieces.

Preheat a frying pan to a medium heat.

Place approximately 10 ml of oil on the frying pan and let it coat the surface.

Slice your brioche or milk bun in half and place the insides on the frying pan to cook until brown, with the bun feeling warm and airy.

Remove your chicken from the deep fryer and allow it to cool on a dripping rack.

THE SAUCE

40 ml of whole egg mayonnaise

½ tsp of chipotle powder

As the chicken cools, prepare your sauce by mixing the ingredients together in a small mixing bowl.

Assemble your sandwich. Eat and enjoy!

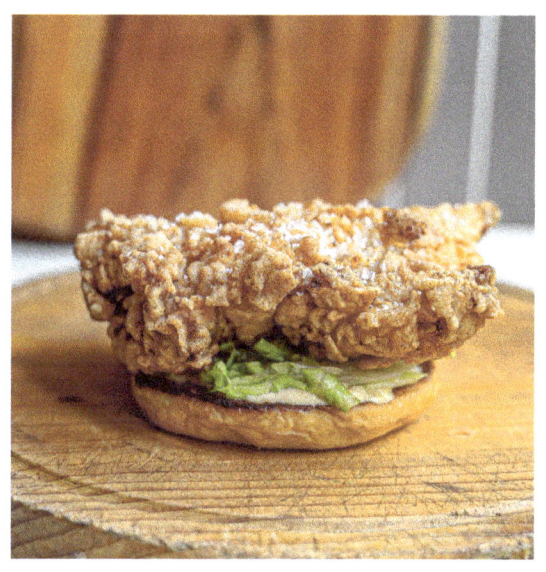
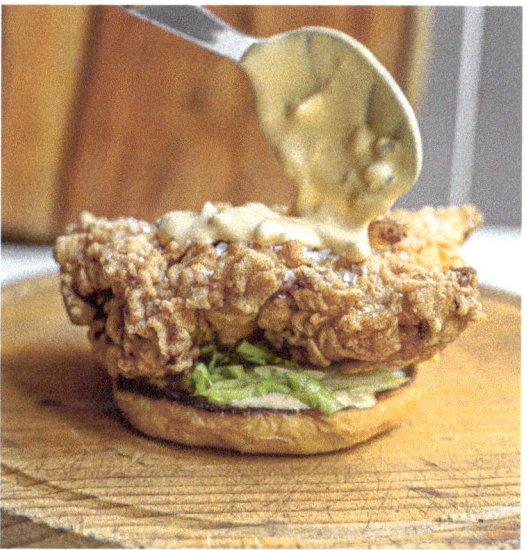

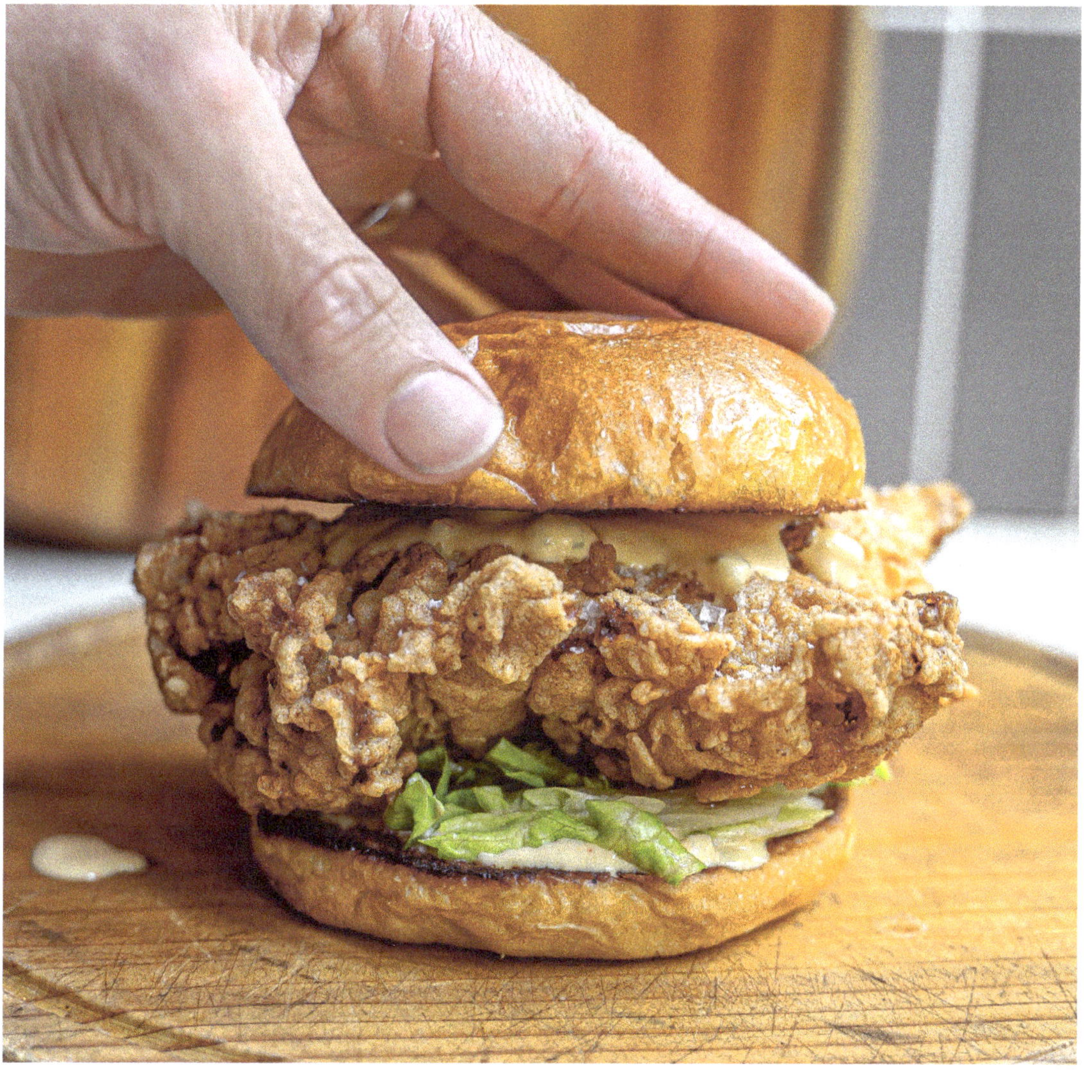

THE SIMPLE SANDO

THE LANDCRUISER

There is something alluring about the Toyota Landcruiser in Australian culture. Watch any movie involving the revered "outback," and, without a doubt, you will see the Landcruiser featured in some part of the movie. When I was growing up, I spent most of a year traveling across Australia in a Toyota Landcruiser with my family. At the young age of five, I was able to truly have the full Australia experience: driving the beast through beachside sand dunes, cooking damper at night, and searching the busy night sky for shooting stars, of which we saw heaps. We drove into the most rural and remote parts of Australia, having showers underneath a plastic bag with holes in it, running into emus, kangaroos, lizards, cassowaries, and nearly being eaten by a saltwater crocodile.

The Landcruiser protected us from all the elements, even as we flew down a dusty highway with bushfires raging on each side as we dodged to avoid the wildlife that was rushing away from danger. The Landcruiser is incredibly reliable; it will never break down, and you can go back to it again and again. But most of all, it's an absolute beast, taking on any terrain that you subject it to. That's what this 4X4 (4 patties x 4 cheese) of a burger is. But, in reality, you could reduce it down to a 2X2. The story just wouldn't have been as cool if I talked about a Hyundai Getz whipping around the harsh Australian outback.

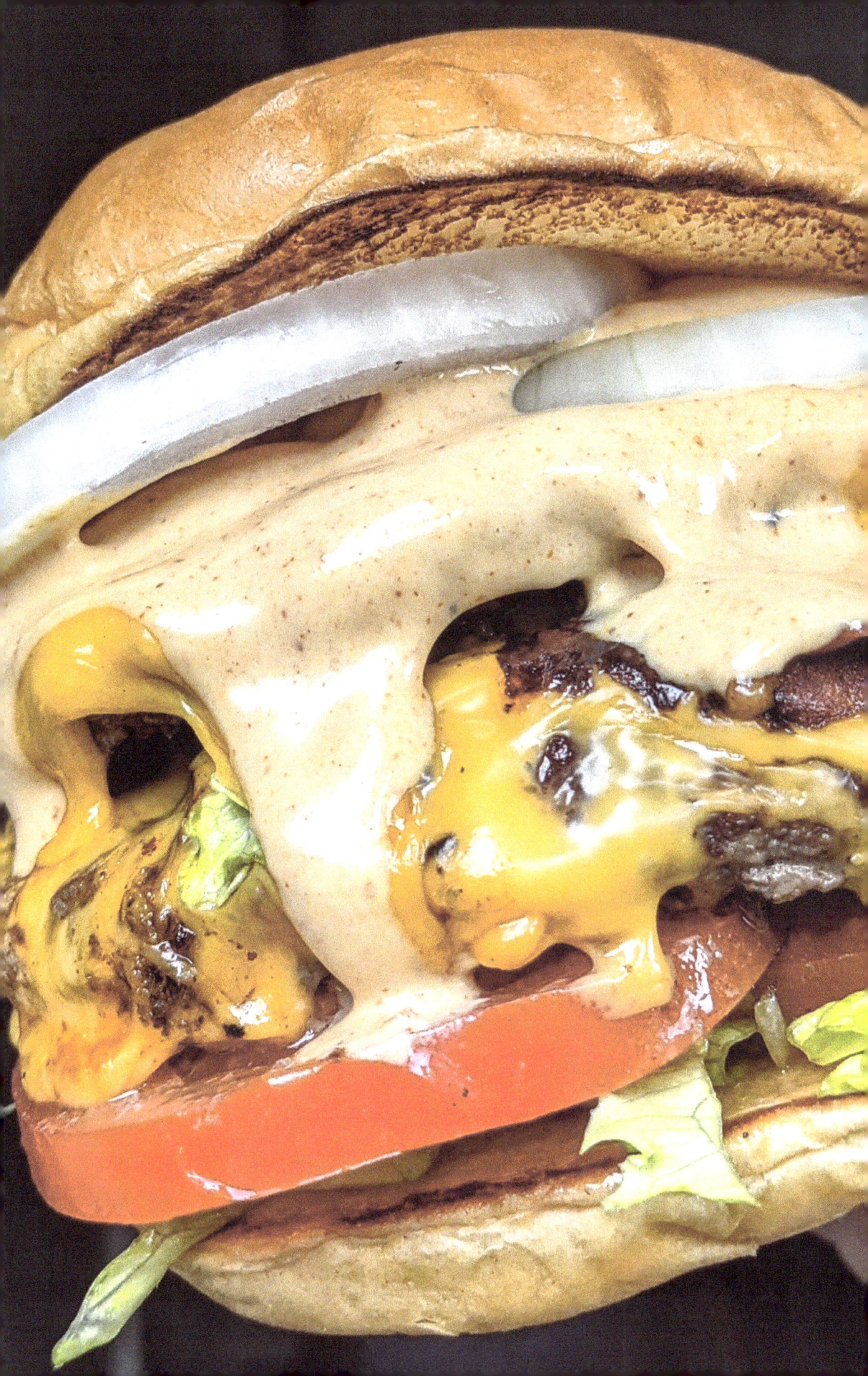

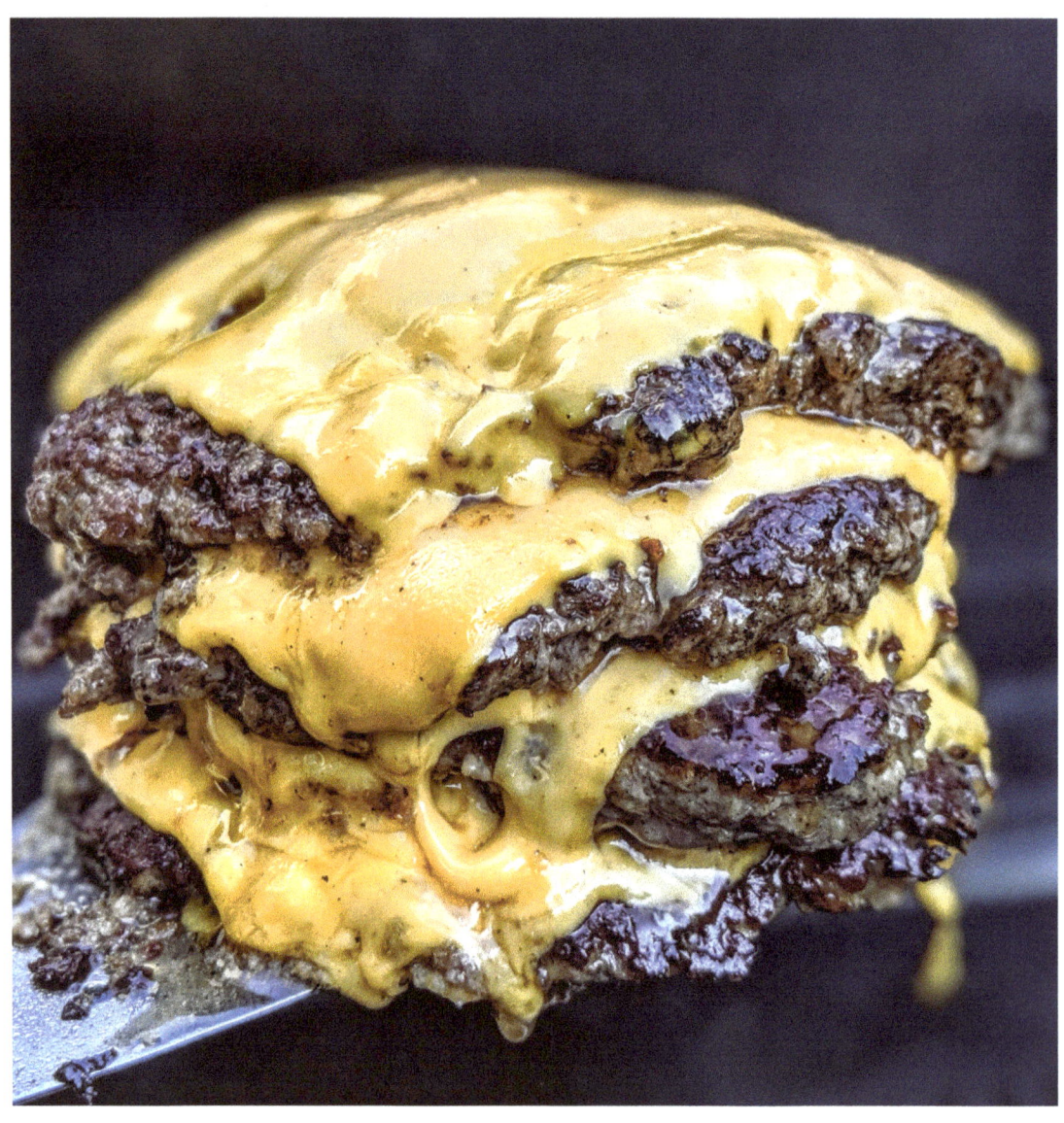

THE SAUCE

40 ml whole egg mayonnaise
20 ml tomato sauce (ketchup)
20 ml mild American mustard
20 ml dill pickle juice
4 pieces of dill pickle (diced)

In a small mixing bowl, place all your sauce ingredients and stir until the sauce is consistent in color and texture. Dice your dill pickle and mix it in with the already-stirred ingredients.

THE BURGER

4 x 80 g balls of beef mince

4 slices of American hi melt cheese

60 ml mild American mustard

2 slices of fresh tomato

40–60 g of diced iceberg lettuce

2–3 rings of white onion

3 x pieces of dill pickle

1 brioche or milk bun

Slice your tomato into thin slices, approximately 3 mm in width. Finely dice your iceberg lettuce. Cut the onion into thin slices, the same size as your tomato, stripping the skin off first. Then remove the inside layers of your onion until it's just the last two. Set all vegetables aside for later assembly.

Slice your brioche/milk bun in half.

Preheat your grill to a medium heat.

Place the inside of your cut buns on the grill, placing a small amount of pressure on them. Wait until they become soft and airy, and slightly brown on the inside. Remove and put aside for assembly.

Heat your grill up to a high temperature, wait until it's smoking hot, and place your patties on the grill one by one, leaving space between them to be flattened out.

Using your preferred smashing tool—you can either opt for a flat smash or an edged smash—press down your patties to just wider than your bun width. After pressing them into the grill, grab your bottle of mild American mustard, apply it to the pink side of the patties in a swirl motion, and wait until the pink has nearly disappeared from the top. Flip your patties and place your hi melt American cheese on top of the cooked/brown side. As soon as the cheese is melted, you can remove the patties from the grill and prepare to assemble your burger.

Assemble your burger with the tomato and lettuce on the bottom bun, patties in the middle, then onion, pickles, and sauce on top of the cooked burgers. Add your top bun and prepare to feast!

Eat and enjoy.

THE STEAK SANDO

This is by far the most requested dish I get asked to make by Mrs. Food Coma. She's obsessed with a good steak sandwich. What a woman. Now, while this is not a burger, just like my fried chicken sando (sandwich in Australian), it is built much like I would construct any other normal burger. The key difference is the protein.

I have to tread carefully whenever I talk about steak or cook it on my Instagram. It's a very personal and subjective dish that most people have an opinion on. They grew up with their dad, grandfather, uncle, aunty, mum, cousin, best friend, and their dog cooking it a certain way, and that's the way it's supposed to be, no ifs, whats, or buts. My way isn't the only way or the highway; it's purely my preferred method for cooking a steak consistently and well. You can do whatever makes you happy and cook your steak to your preferred doneness. The most important thing is that you enjoy your steak sando. Say it with me, "Staayyyk sand-ohhhhhhh."

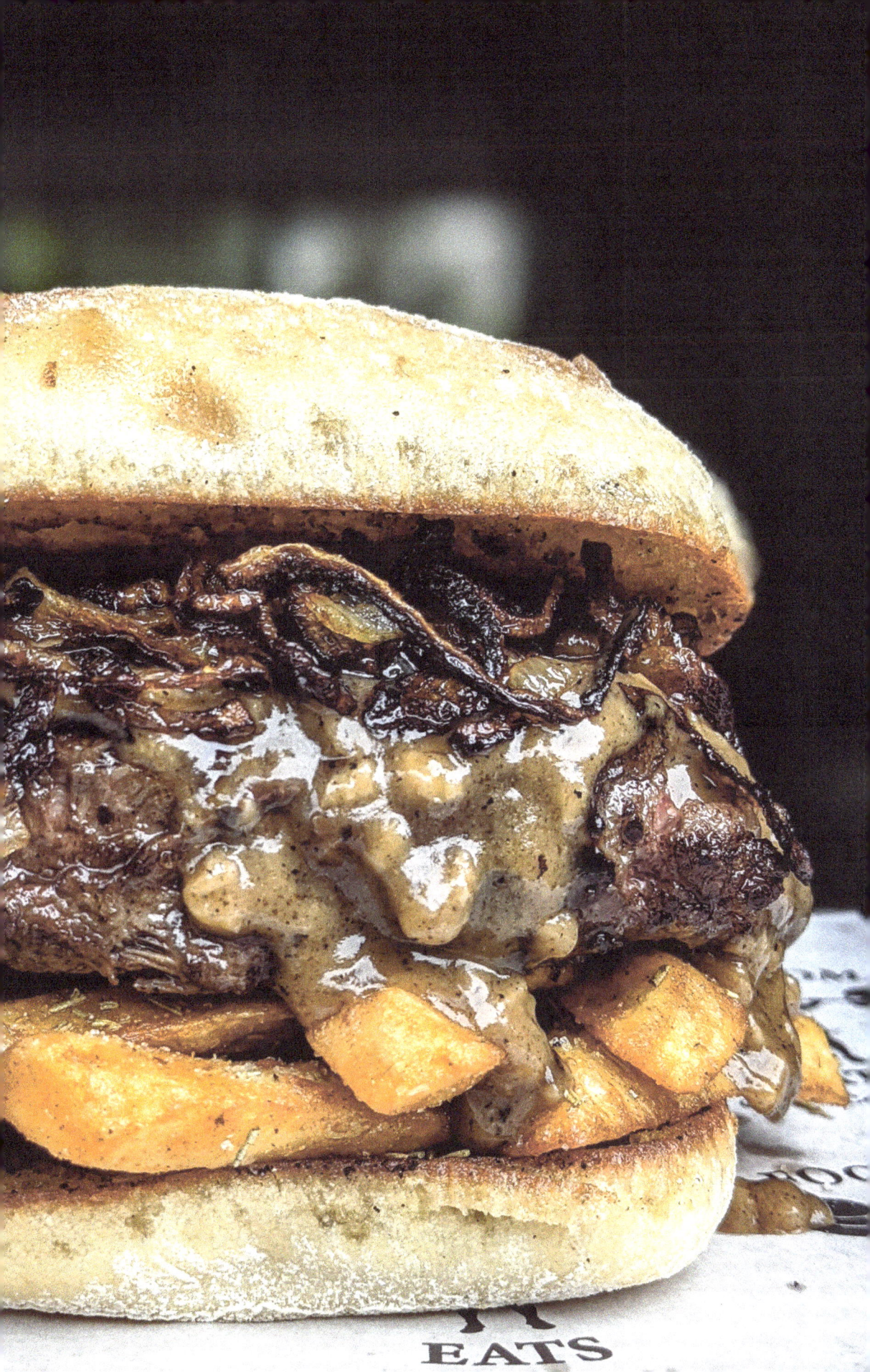

FOOD COMA STEAK COOKING TIPS

» Find yourself a great butcher that has a consistent product and understands their product well. They will be able to assist you in finding the right steak for the right occasion and will often offer you tips on how to cook it.

» Be wary of fat content. A scotch fillet steak will cook very differently to an eye fillet. One will need a bit more exterior assistance in the caramelization process through added oil or butter. I'm looking at you, eye fillet.

» Steak thickness will very heavily affect how long you cook the steak for. There's not one perfect amount of time for any steak. A thicker steak, while great for getting a nice, rare finished product, may sometimes burn or overcook on the exterior before the inside is cooked to the desired doneness. You can avoid this by opting for a medium heat for the entire cook, reverse searing, finishing it in the oven, or—and bear with me on this one—regularly turning it. There's more than one way to skin a cat, or cook a steak in this instance, and all can be effective. A thinner steak will need an incredibly hard and fast approach. A screaming-hot cast-iron pan will do the trick, with a small amount of oil to aid it in its caramelization journey.

» Find yourself a bargain. Just because you *can* pay $100 per kilogram for a steak doesn't always mean you have to. If you're careful and pay very close attention to products in your local supermarket, sometimes you can find an absolute steal of a steak. Be wary of fat marbling—that's one of the most important factors of what constitutes a costly steak. If you see something with some serious marbling sitting on the shelf of your local supermarket, it's totally appropriate to shoulder charge Grandma out of the way to claim your prize.

» If in doubt, go the highest heat for your grill or frying pan. Do you know what's worse than a burned steak that's too rare in the middle for your liking? A boiled, gray steak. It reminds me of those rubbery, shoe-like minute steaks you'd get on a cruise. I'd much rather caramelize the outside of my steak and finish it in the oven to achieve desired rareness than deal with any sort of gray steak barely clinging to life.

» Let the steak reach room temperature before cooking.

» Pat down your steak with a paper towel before you apply your seasoning. One of the biggest factors stopping your steak from reaching peak caramelization is the liquid on the outside (myoglobin). When it first hits the grill, it will do two things: it will steam, and it will cool down the grill and create a pool of liquid around your steak. Save yourself the hassle of trying to counteract this with the hottest grill in the world. Just wipe the steak dry.

» Play around with flavored butters. There is nothing more beautiful than basting a piece of rested steak with flavored butter. It feels like you're giving your steak that last little massage, willing it toward tenderness and allowing its muscles to soak in every flavor you put in the butter. This favors people with a gas stove and while it's not impossible to achieve on induction, it's pretty damn difficult.

» Don't feel the need to overcomplicate your steak's flavor, but don't you *ever* forget to season it. Even if it's just a few pinches of sea salt flakes, you truly bring meat alive when you season and cook it.

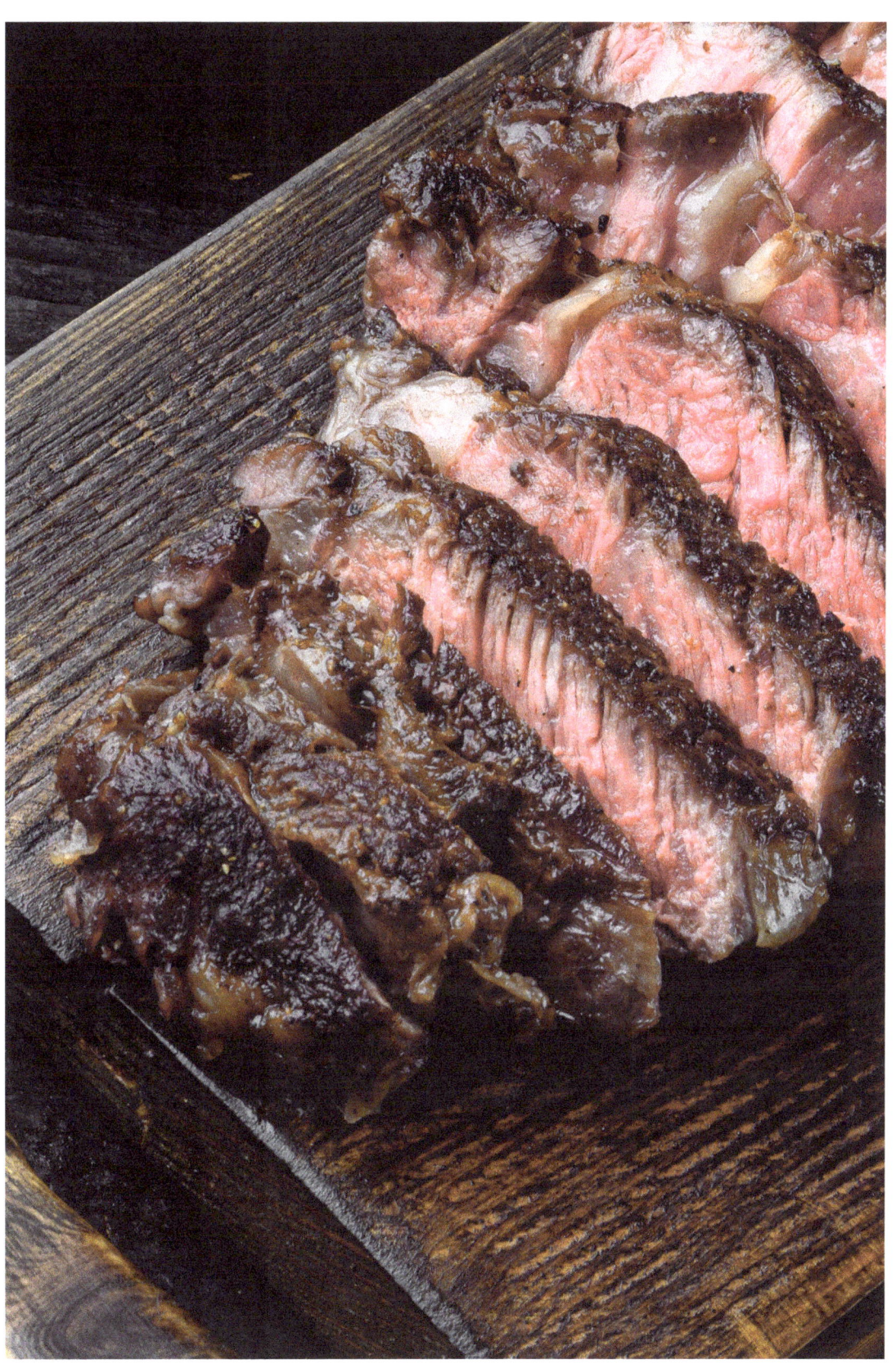

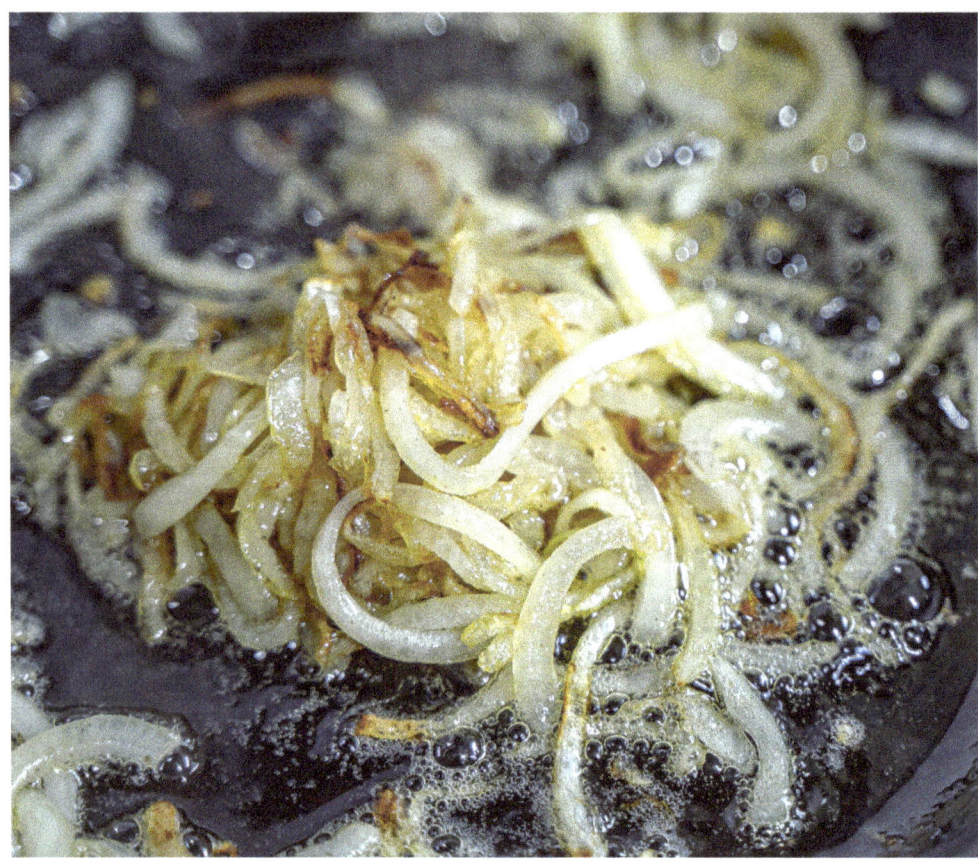

A SIMPLE PEPPER SAUCE

2 tbsp of butter
2 tbsp of plain flour
1 ¼ cups of thickened cream
1–2 tsp of salt flakes
1 tsp of ground black pepper
1 tsp of coarsely ground pepper
½ tsp of garlic powder
½ tsp of onion powder

For your steak sandwich, you can use a simple pepper sauce. Here's a quick crash course.

Melt the butter in a nonstick pan on a medium heat.

Stir your butter as you put the plain flour in the pan. Whisk at the end until the consistency is smooth.

Add your dry ingredients, slowly stirring for approximately 3–4 minutes until mixed in.

Place the thickened cream into the pan and slowly stir until the mixture thickens.

Put on a low heat until thickened to desired consistency.

NOW BACK TO COOKING THE SANDO...

1 medium brown onion, sliced
40 g of salted butter
10 ml of canola oil
100 g of steak-cut fries
150–250 g scotch fillet steak
1 tsp of fresh or dried rosemary
1 tsp of salt flakes
A simple pepper sauce
1 ciabatta roll

Heat up a frying pan to a medium heat and melt your salted butter. While the butter is melting, prepare your onions by peeling and slicing them into half-circle slivers.

Place the sliced onion into the melted butter and mix until all the onion is broken apart. Stir every 30 seconds until the onion is caramelized and brown.

Remove fried onion from the frying pan and place aside for later assembly. Slice your ciabatta roll in half and place the insides of the buns in the onion-flavored butter, cooking until brown.

Preheat your deep fryer to 180°C (356°F).

Prepare your scotch fillet steak by patting it down with a tea towel until dry on the exterior. Grab a pinch of salt flakes for each side of the steak and season evenly. Allow it to sit for 5–10 minutes while you heat up your frying pan.

Heat your stainless steel or cast-iron frying pan to a high heat. While your frying pan is heating up, place your steak-cut fries into the deep fryer and cook until golden brown.

Lightly oil the pan. Place your seasoned scotch fillet steak on the hot frying pan and sear until the exterior is brown and caramelized, then flip and repeat on the other side. Finish in the oven or continue flipping every 30–40 seconds until your steak has reached preferred doneness. The best way to check is to get an instant-read meat probe and check the interior temperature. There are a few sources online that will tell you the guidelines for internal temperature in your country.

Remove steak from the frying pan and allow to rest for at least 4–6 minutes. While your steak is resting, season your fries by placing them in a large mixing bowl and mixing them with the rosemary and salt. Season to your preference.

Assemble all your ingredients together in the ciabatta roll with a simple pepper sauce.

Eat and enjoy!

THE GODFATHER

Some of you may or may not know, but I was *this* close to ending up on My Kitchen Rules. Yep, and what a TV diva I would have been. The lovely Mrs. Food Coma and I did all the auditions, to the point that we even had a film crew at her house to do a trial run. It all seemed to be going smoothly, but they decided to change the direction of the show. Part of me wonders how we'd do on a show like that. We are both incredibly competitive and have an obsession with food. However, the drama side of the show may not have been a great color on us. While I'm generally a nice guy, if you put me in a competitive environment, I become an absolute monster. I don't think that would have boded well for our "characters." Nevertheless, we had a ton of fun in the auditioning process, and it opened our eyes to what could have been.

Instead, I took the opportunity to concentrate on my business, help grow brands, and cook even more. The whole story here—and believe me, I'm getting there—is that this burger is what I cooked up in our audition for the show. I was pretty proud of it. This burger will always have a place in my life—and a delicious place that is. I hope you will enjoy it as well.

For this recipe, it's optional whether you want to make your own mayonnaise, which is what I did for the audition. I'll also give you a crash course garlic mayo that's a couple steps quicker.

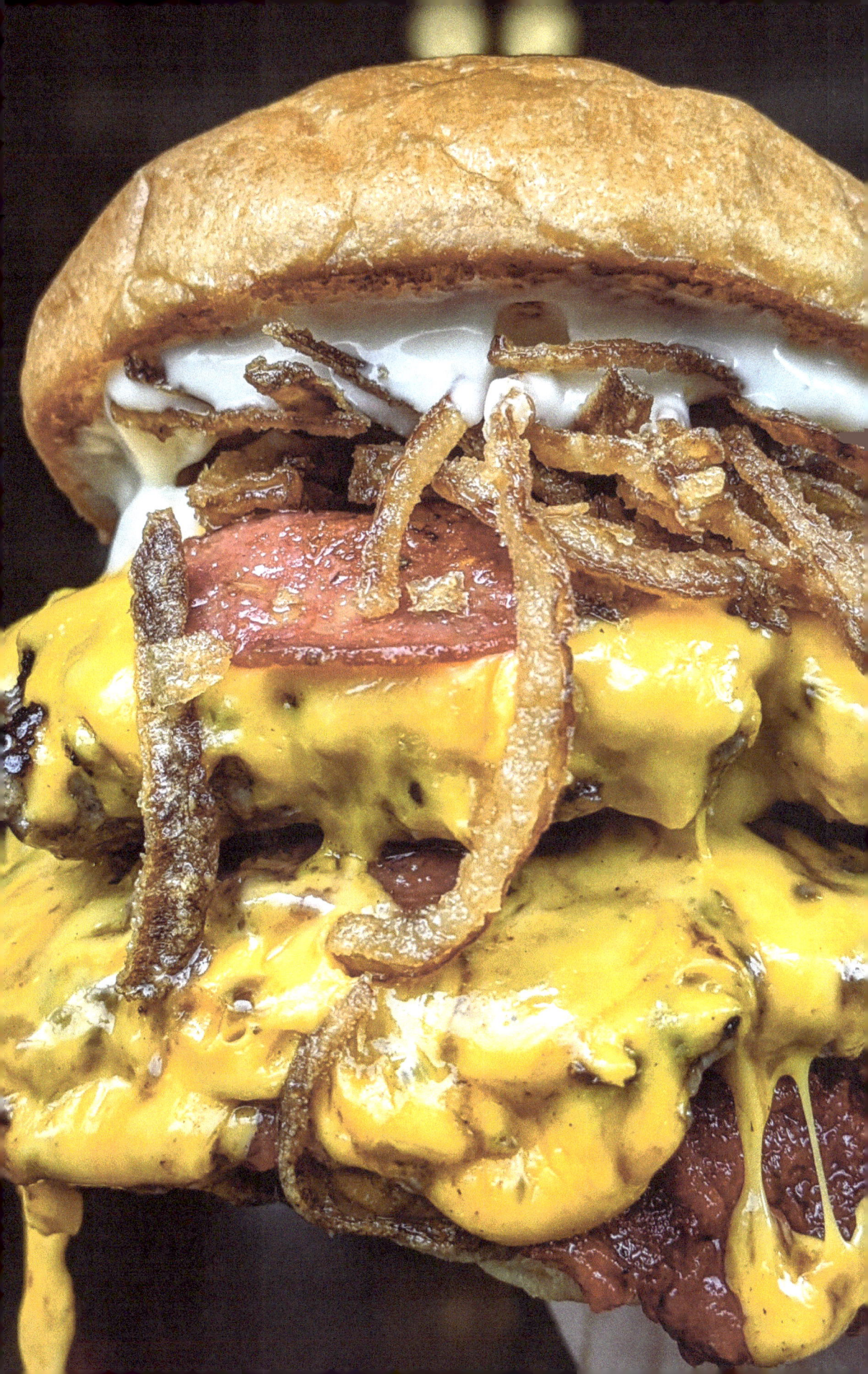

A REALLY SIMPLE GARLIC MAYO

500 ml of whole egg mayonnaise

A whole head of garlic

20 ml of canola oil

Slice the top off the head of garlic, exposing the tops of all the cloves.

Place on a tray with baking paper underneath and apply the canola oil to the exposed cloves.

Heat your oven to 180°C (356°F) and place the head of garlic in the oven, clove side up, and cook until brown and soft.

Remove the cloves from the head with a fork.

Place cooked garlic into the whole egg mayonnaise and blitz with a food processor until smooth and consistent.

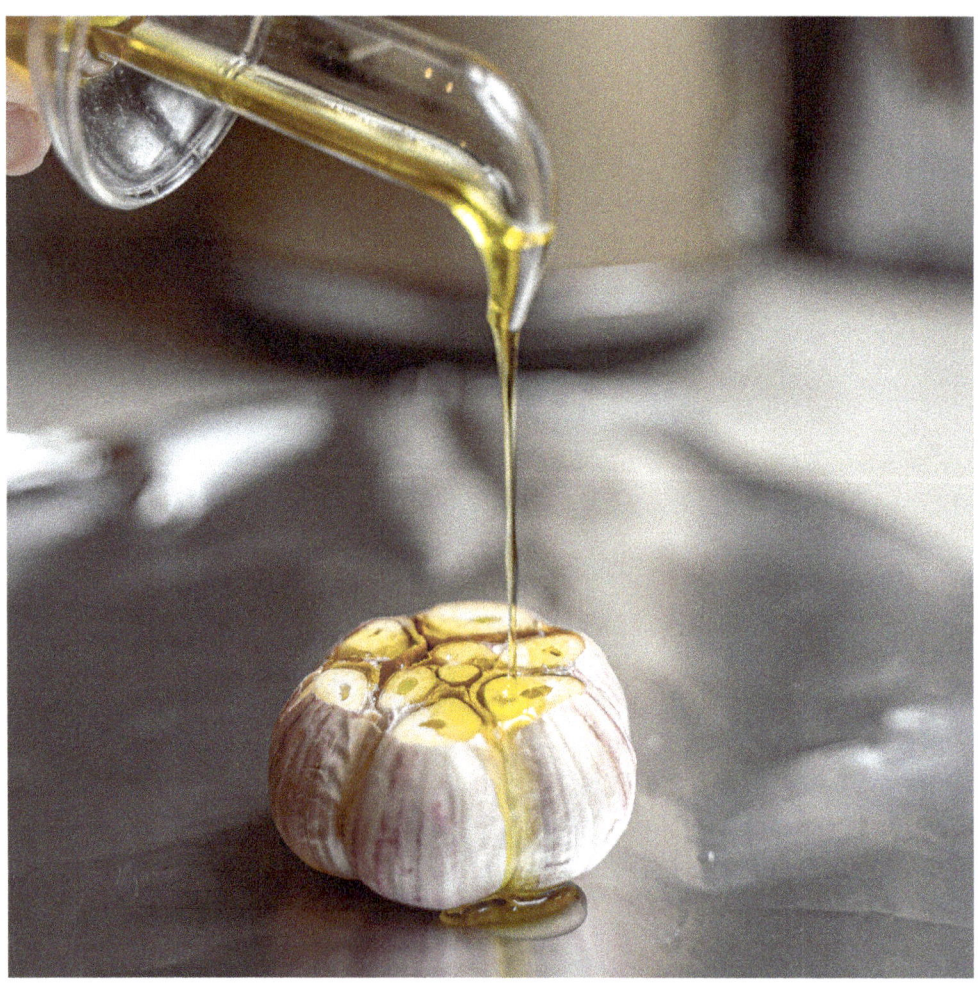

THE BURGER

6 slices of pepperoni

Half an onion, sliced

1 cup of plain flour

2 x 150 g balls of beef mince

2 slices of American hi melt cheese

1 brioche or milk bun

1 tbsp of **a REALLY simple garlic mayo**

1 tbsp of your favorite pizza sauce

Salt flakes

Slice your onion into half circle slivers, approximately 2 mm in thickness.

Place your flour into a medium-sized mixing bowl. Toss your onion in the flour until lightly coated.

Heat your deep fryer to 170°C (338°F). Cook the floured onion until golden brown and crunchy.

Lightly season and toss the crispy onion in a large mixing bowl.

Place your sliced pepperoni into a cast-iron pan and grill at a medium heat until crispy, flipping halfway through. Remove and set aside when cooking the burger.

Slice your brioche/milk bun in half.

Preheat your grill to a medium heat.

Place the inside of your cut buns on the grill, placing a small amount of pressure on them. Wait until they become soft and airy, and slightly brown on the inside. Remove and put aside for assembly.

Heat your grill up to a high temperature, wait until it's smoking hot, and place your patties on the grill one by one, leaving space between them to be flattened out.

Using your preferred smashing tool—you can either opt for a flat smash or an edged smash—press down your patties to just wider than your bun width. After pressing them into the grill, season with salt flakes evenly on each patty and wait until the pink has nearly disappeared from the top. Flip your patties and place your hi melt American cheese on top of the cooked/brown side, then place your cooked pepperoni on both patties. As soon as the cheese is melted, you can remove the patties from the grill and prepare to assemble your burger.

Eat and enjoy!

THE GODFATHER

THE JUICY LUCY

The humble Juicy Lucy has been a part of the burger world for quite some time. For those who don't know who our friend Lucy is, she's a delicious, cheese-stuffed, gooey, and *juicy* burger. The origin of this cool burger is still uncertain. Some people claim that it came from Matt's Bar, others that it was from 5-8 Club, both in Minneapolis. Either way, hats off to you, whoever you are that birthed the juicy Lucy.

I was tossing up whether I'd include this recipe in the book. But as with the Oklahoma Smash Burger and the Homer Simpson, it's as important to me to show off the world of cool burgers as it is to show my own. At the end of the day, with every burger I make, I have no doubt that someone else's version already exists somewhere. But rather than argue about whose burger is better or who was first—definitely not me—I want to celebrate what makes burgers awesome. So, without further ado, here's my interpretation of a very simple Juicy Lucy.

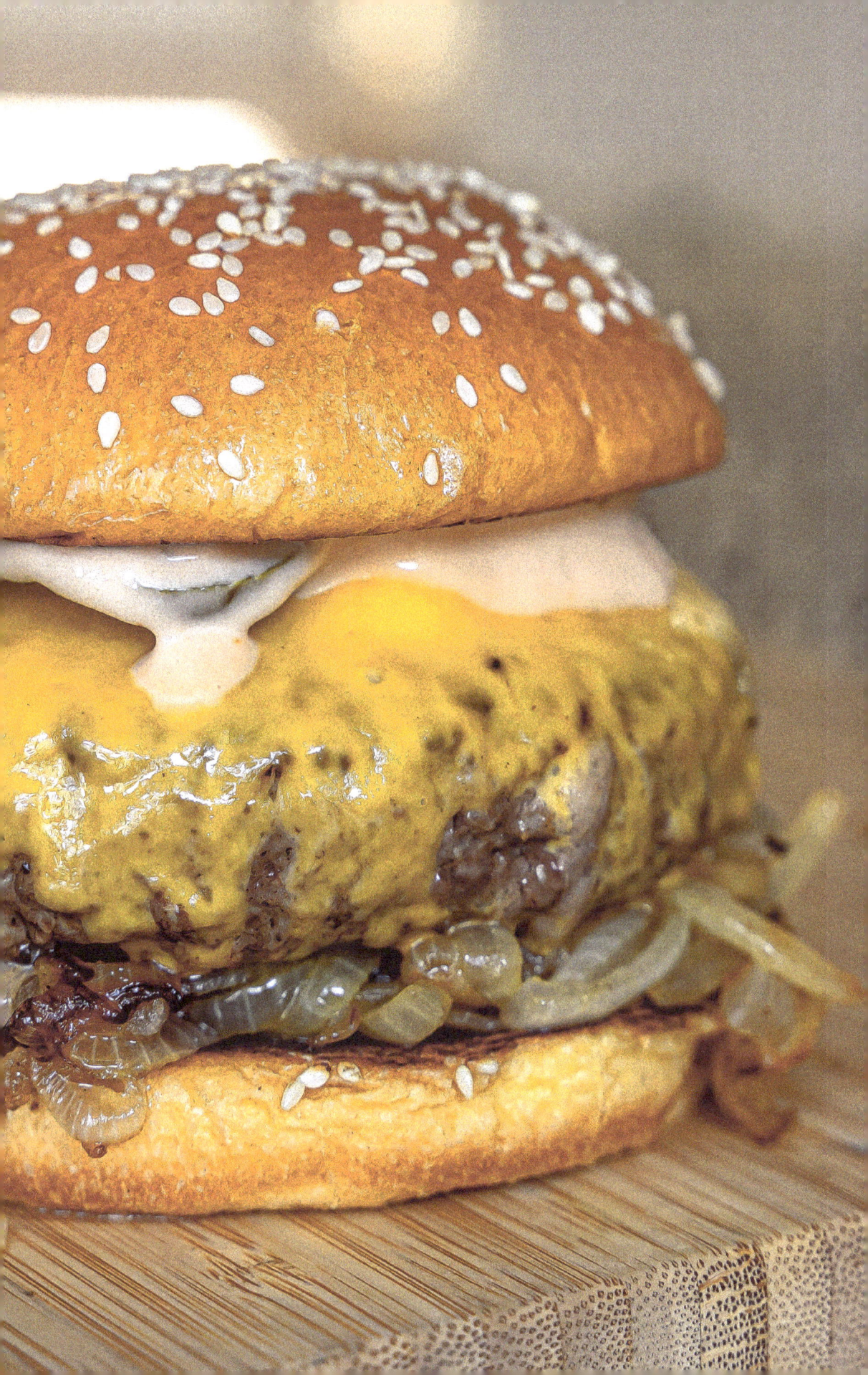

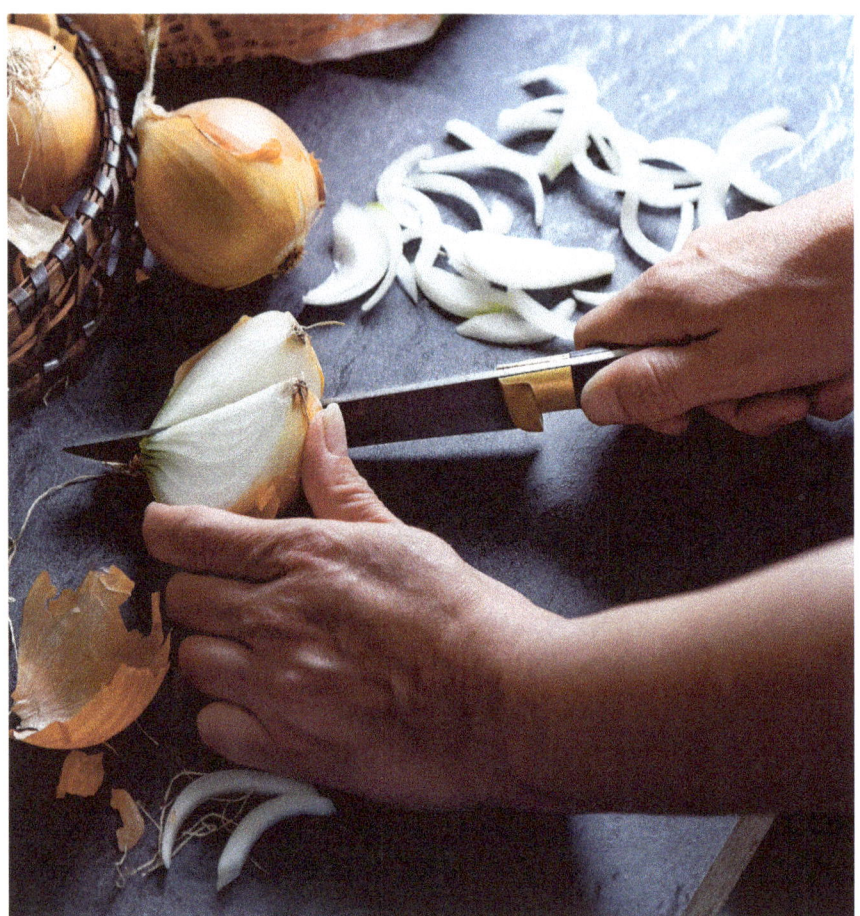

A SIMPLE ONION JAM

2 large brown onions
50 g salted butter
2 tbsp of brown sugar
¼ cup of balsamic vinegar
1 tsp of chili powder
1 tsp of smoked paprika

Peel and slice your onion into half-circle slivers, approximately 2 mm thick.

Heat a frying pan to a medium heat and melt your butter.

Cook your onions in the butter until brown and caramelized.

Add brown sugar, balsamic vinegar, chili powder, and smoked paprika.

Stir until mixed in, then reduce to a low heat.

Leave to thicken, stirring every minute until desired consistency (I like mine extra thiccc).

Store in the fridge until needed.

THE SAUCE

40 ml of whole egg mayonnaise

20 ml of tomato sauce (ketchup)

20 ml of American mild mustard

30 ml of dill pickle juice

15 g of diced dill pickles

½ tsp of chili powder

Combine your sauce ingredients in a small mixing bowl and stir with a spoon until fully mixed in.

THE BURGER

2 x 125 g balls of beef mince

2 slices of American hi melt cheese

40 g of shredded mozzarella (or your cheese of choice)

1 brioche or milk bun

30 g of caramelized onion jam (for homemade, see *a simple onion jam*)

Salt flakes

Prepare your Juicy Lucy patty by flattening your balls of mince between two pieces of baking paper until 2 cm wider than your bun. Place your shredded mozzarella on one of your patties and place the other patty on top. Proceed to join the two patties together until the cheese is fully sealed between them.

Slice your brioche or milk bun in half.

Heat your frying pan to a medium temperature and place the two insides of the buns on the pan and remove when lightly brown.

Season both sides of your Juicy Lucy patty with salt flakes.

Leave your frying pan on a medium heat and cook your Juicy Lucy. Depending on the thickness of the patty, cook for 2–4 minutes on each side.

Once the Juicy Lucy patty is fully caramelized, place your American hi melt cheese on top and cover with a lid until melted. This should also finish cooking the inside of the patty.

Remove from the frying pan and allow to rest for 4 minutes. Assemble your burger with your caramelized onion jam, Juicy Lucy patty, special sauce, and bun.

Eat and enjoy!

THE 4:20 O'CLOCK

Look, let's not be naive here. Most people, thanks to popular culture, understand the reference 4:20. So many movies are not only inspired by 4:20, but completely based on it: Super Troopers, Pineapple Express, The Gentlemen, We're the Millers, and basically any movie featuring Seth Rogan, just to name a few. Stoner references, even given to us at a young age—I'm looking at you Scooby Doo and Shaggy—are everywhere in pop culture. With all the movies that give the nod to marijuana, most of us know about "the munchies." I am in no way a stoner, but damn, my mind definitely works like one when I'm thinking about food. So, it's my turn to jump on the bandwagon and provide you with a drool-inducing stoner's love affair of a burger.

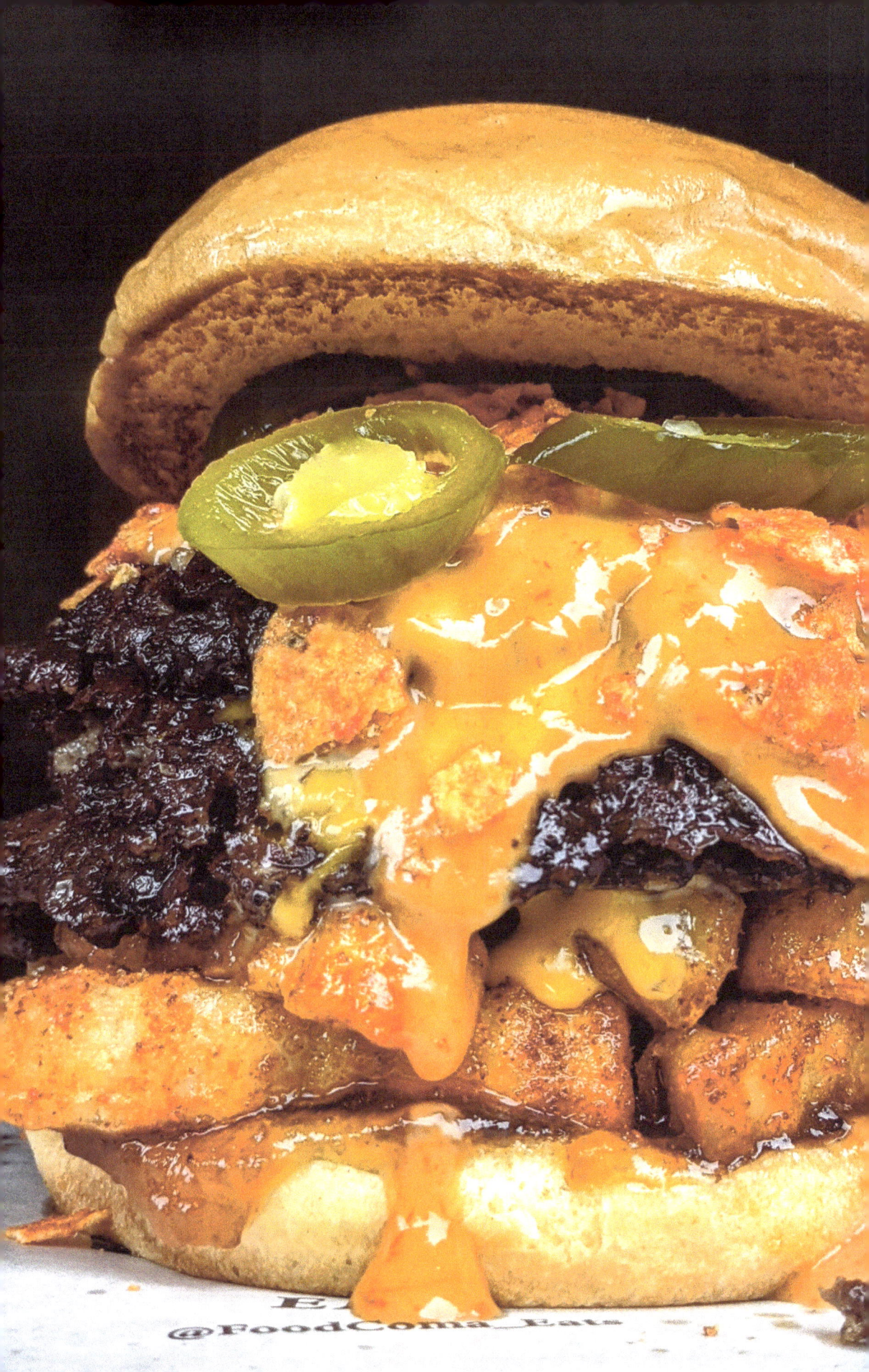

THE SAUCE

20 ml of sriracha hot sauce
20 ml maple syrup
40 ml of whole egg mayonnaise

In a small bowl, mix all your sauce ingredients together until smooth and consistent.

THE BURGER

¼ cup of crushed Doritos
1 cup of crinkle-cut fries
1 tsp of smoked paprika
1 tsp of salt flakes
1–3 x 100 g balls of beef mince
1–3 slices of American hi melt cheese
20 g of pickled jalapeños
1 brioche or milk bun
1 tbsp of *a simple onion jam*

Heat up your deep fryer to 180°C (356°F) and cook your crinkle-cut fries until golden brown.

Season your fries with the smoked paprika and salt flakes. Leave in the oven on a low temp until ready to assemble.

Slice your brioche/milk bun in half.

Preheat your grill to a medium heat.

Place the inside of your cut buns on the grill, placing a small amount of pressure on them. Wait until they become soft and airy, and slightly brown on the inside. Remove and put aside for assembly.

Heat your grill up to a high temperature, wait until it's smoking hot, and place your patties on the grill one by one, leaving space between them to be flattened out.

Using your preferred smashing tool—you can either opt for a flat smash or an edged smash—press down your patties to just wider than your bun width. After pressing them into the grill, season each patty evenly with salt flakes and wait until the pink has nearly disappeared from the top. Flip your patties and place your hi melt American cheese on top of the cooked/brown side. As soon as the cheese is melted, you can remove the patties from the grill and prepare to assemble your burger.

Assemble your burger with the leftover ingredients, your cooked patties, and the seasoned fries.

Eat and enjoy!

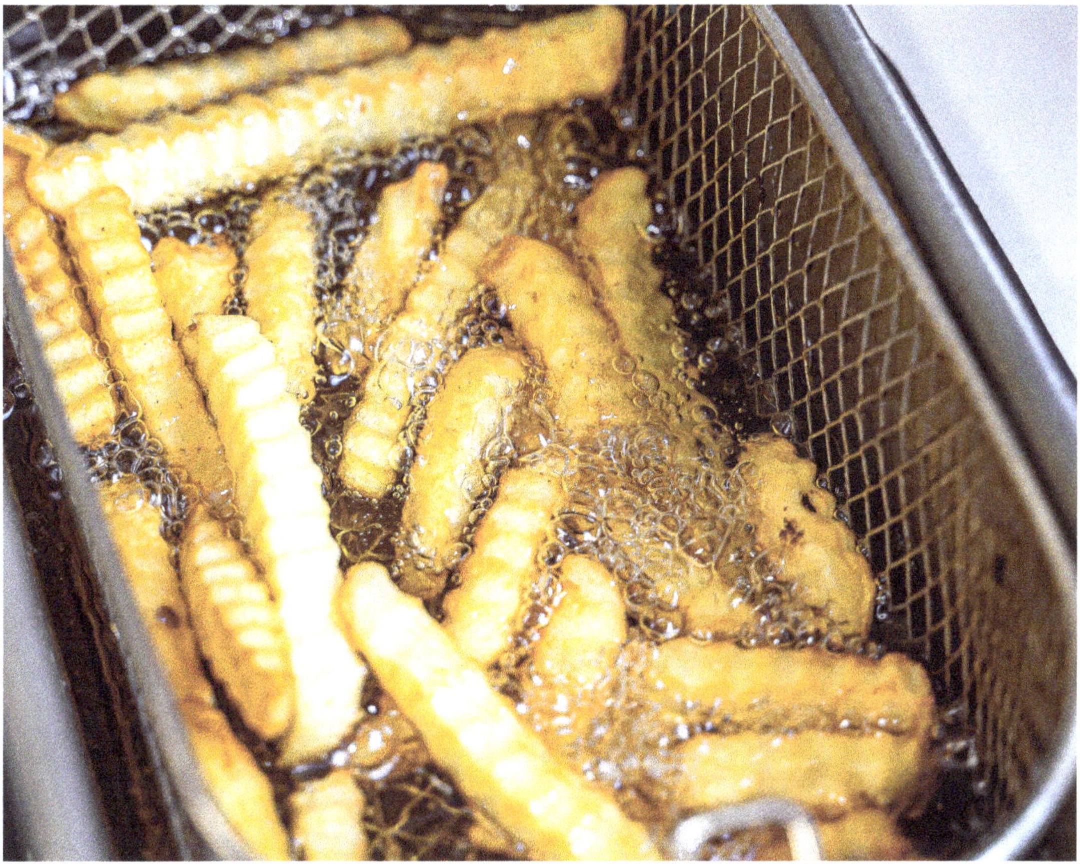

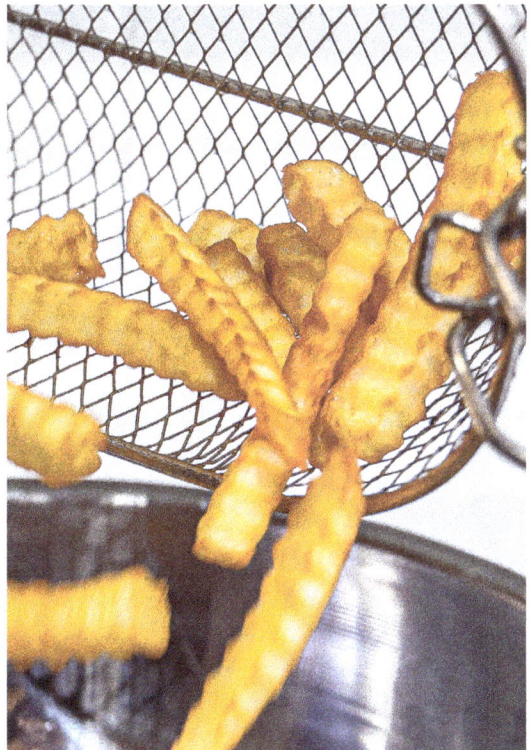
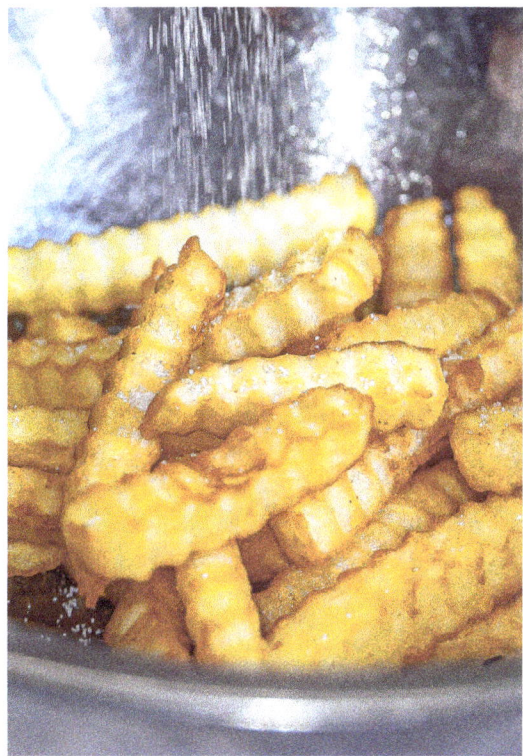

THE TRIPLE BYPASS

Almost every burger joint in Sydney either has their version of this burger or has had it on their menu. It usually has names such as "Big Daddy," "The Monster," "Heart Attack," "Bic Boi," or "The Undertaker" and often means you're in for a heart-stopping, artery-clogging, cholesterol-injecting experience of a burger. As a little, naive, burger fanboy, I traveled around Sydney in search of their biggest and baddest burgers.

Eventually I entered the territory of burgers that were so horribly large and calorie-ridden, they almost weren't even burgers anymore. That's where my competitive eating career really took off. I went from dieting strictly six days a week—because Saturdays are for the boys—to having one huge, eye popping, ten to fifteen patty burger a week. Of course, I had to make adjustments to my life to fit this in, so I was intermittent fasting every day and finishing most sessions at the gym completely spent, with my face a pale white from cardiovascular and muscular stress. These burgers are what started my competitive eating career, so they will always hold a special place in my heart (and arteries). So, here's my own version for you to make from home to release the competitive eater in you.

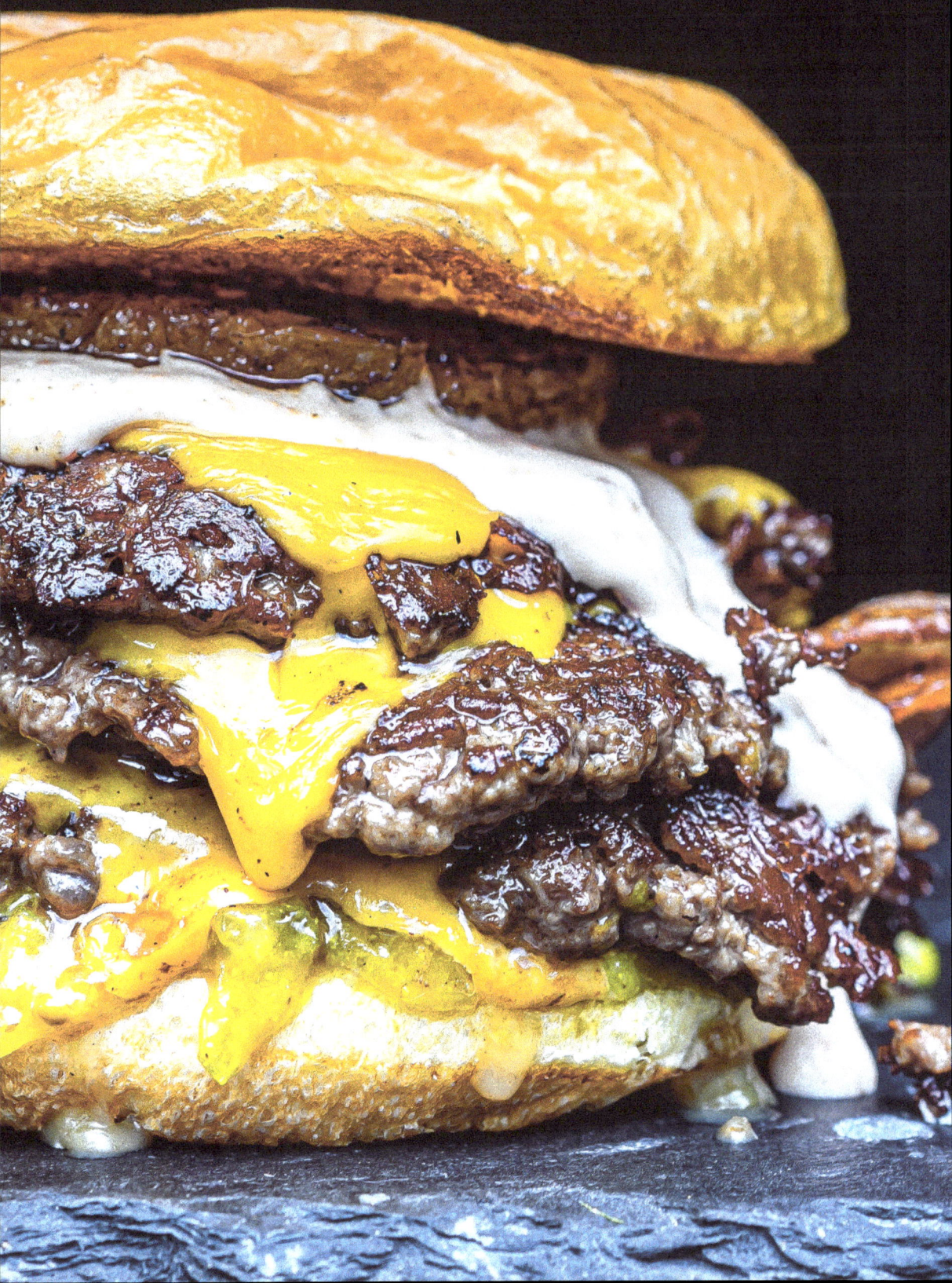

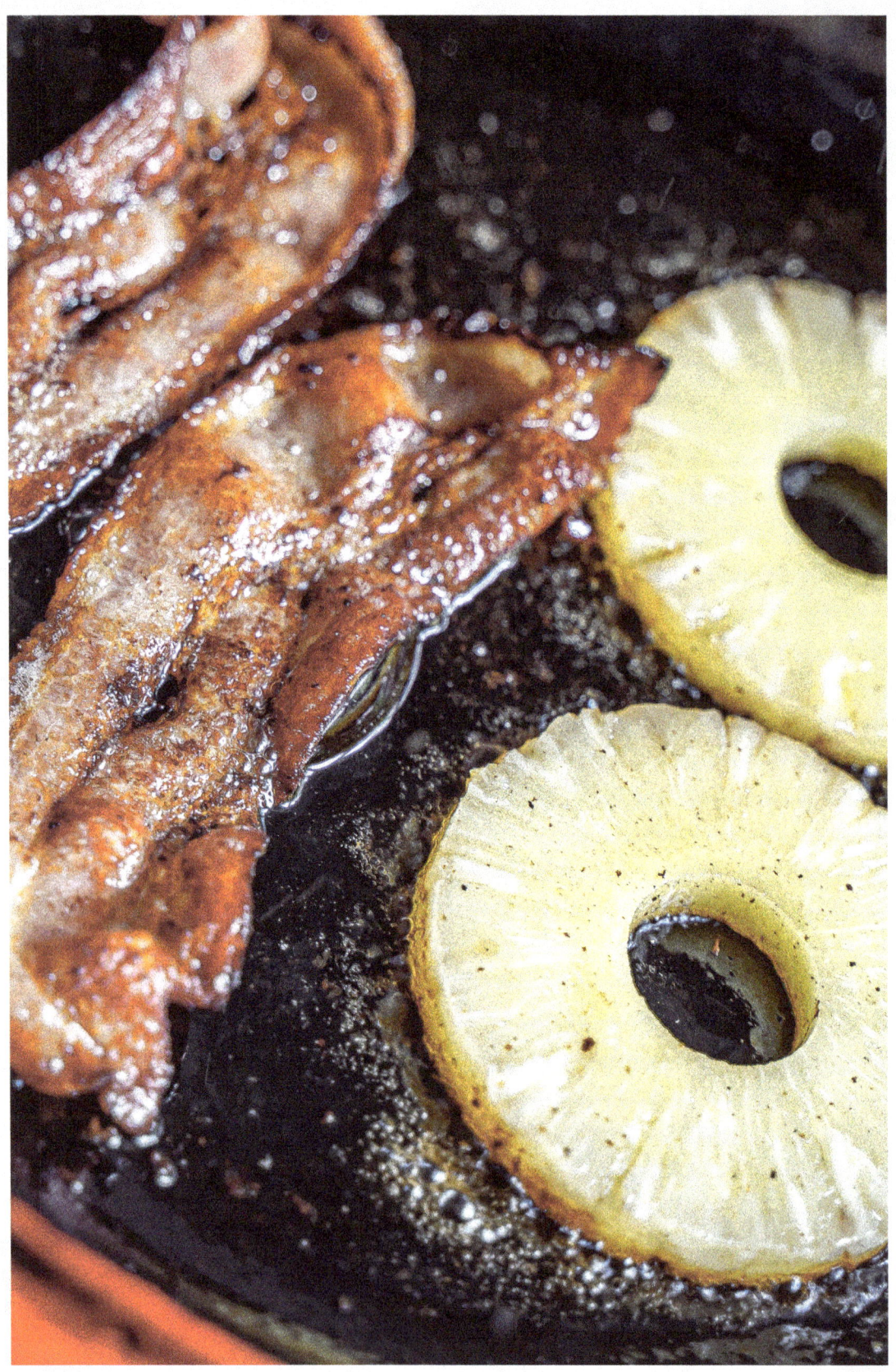

THE SAUCE

20 ml of Byron Bay Chilli Co. mango habanero hot sauce (or a similar alternative)

30 ml of whole egg mayonnaise

In a small bowl, mix your mango habanero hot sauce and whole egg mayonnaise together until smooth and consistent.

THE BURGER

1 tbsp of pickle relish

3 x 120 g balls of beef mince

3 slices of American hi melt cheese

3 rashers of Black Forest streaky bacon (or a similar alternative)

1 slice of canned pineapple

Salt flakes

1 brioche or milk bun

Slice your brioche/milk bun in half

Preheat your grill to a medium heat

Place the inside of your cut buns on the grill, placing a small amount of pressure on them. Wait until they become soft and airy, and slightly brown on the inside. Remove and put aside for assembly.

Heat your grill up to a high temperature, wait until it's smoking hot, and place your patties on the grill one by one, leaving space between them to be flattened out.

Using your preferred smashing tool—you can either opt for a flat smash or an edged smash—press down your patties to just wider than your bun width.

In the remaining space on your grill, place your bacon and pineapple.

After pressing the patties into the grill and placing down your bacon/pineapple, season the patties with salt flakes evenly and wait until the pink has nearly disappeared from the top. Flip your patties, bacon, and pineapple and place your hi melt American cheese on top of the cooked/brown side of the patties. As soon as the cheese is melted, place the cooked bacon on top of each patty, stack them, and finish with the pineapple on top. Now you can remove the patties from the grill and prepare to assemble your burger.

Eat and enjoy!

THE MONSTER MASH

I struggled incredibly hard trying to give meaning to this sandwich. In all reality, it could be a homage to 420, mi goreng, or even a Pringle fried chicken recipe. You could pick one of these ingredients and use it as a hero item in any normal burger, whether it's the mi goreng mayo or the Pringle fried chicken, and it would be cool enough on its own. This sandwich is the Frankenstein's monster of all my recipes in one freakish, scary, and oddly delicious meal. Like all good things mashed together, each part of the recipe has its place and is there for a reason.

However, this burger doesn't have a particular theme attached to it. It's almost the outcast, the one I kept in the basement when friends came over but, like the Hunchback of Notre Dame, was a pretty alright sandwich once you got to know it. Yep, I'm going to go with that. There's your theme.

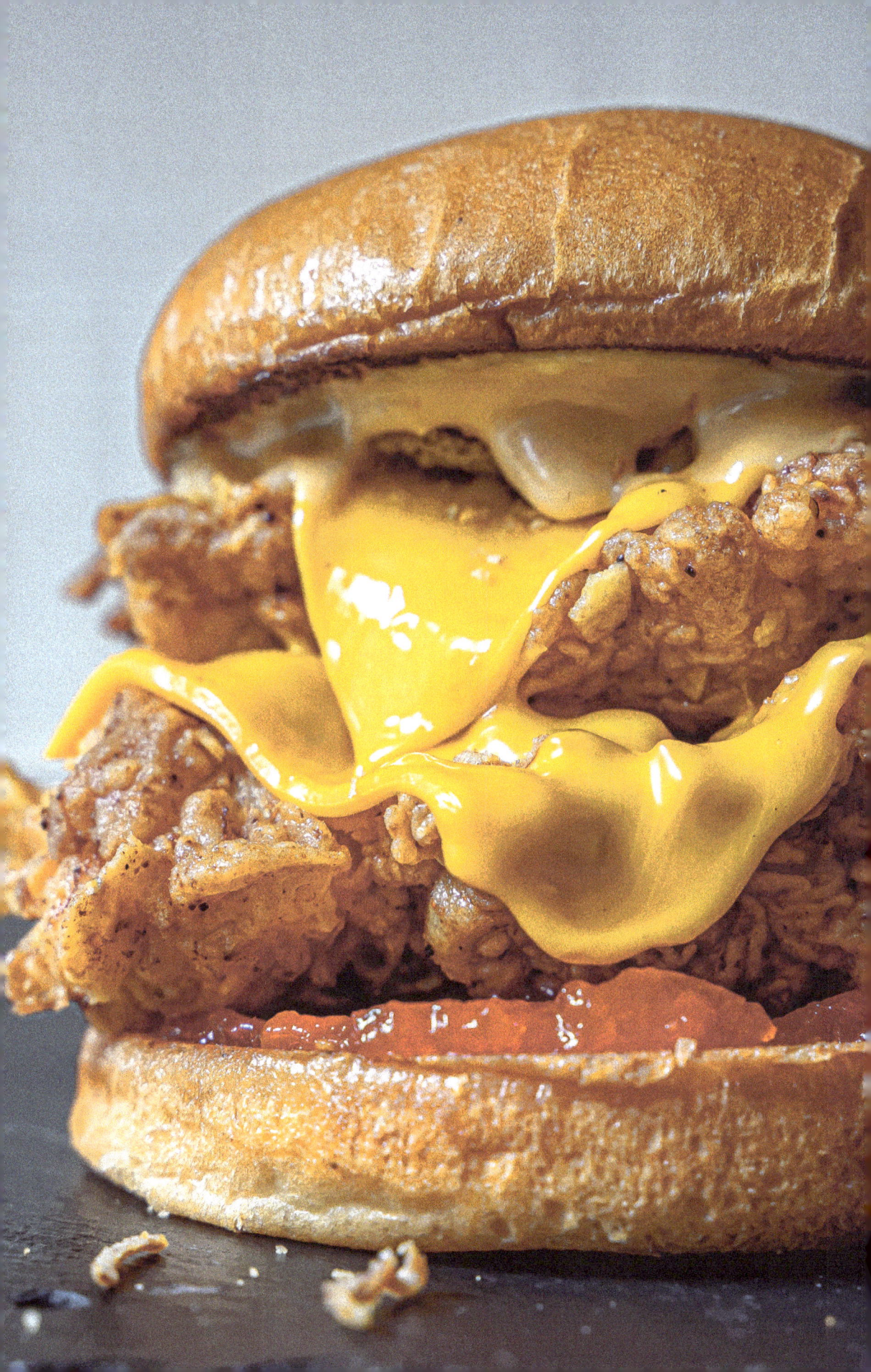

THE SAUCE

1 mi goreng flavor packet

60 ml of whole egg mayonnaise

Mix the sauce ingredients together in a small bowl until the mixture is smooth and consistent.

THE PRINGLE FRIED CHICKEN

1 cup of crushed Pringles

¾ cup of plain flour

¾ cup of corn flour

1 tsp of ground white pepper

1 tsp of coarsely ground black pepper

1 tsp of smoked paprika

1 tsp of chili powder

1 tsp of onion powder

1 tsp of garlic powder

200 ml of buttermilk

150–200 g chicken thigh

Following the steps in **Food Coma Fried Chicken Hot Tips** on page 86, prepare your chicken either overnight in a buttermilk brine or plain flour then buttermilk.

Place all the dry ingredients for the Pringle fried chicken in a large bowl and mix with a whisk until all the flour and spice clumps are gone. There should be 3–4 mm pieces of crushed Pringles throughout the mixture.

Remove the chicken thigh from the buttermilk and mix into the Pringle fried chicken flour. Be sure to coat both sides of the fillet, applying a small amount of pressure to stick the flour to the buttermilk. Remove from the flour and give it a small shake to dislodge any loose bits. Feel free to apply a second buttermilk and flour dredge; however, this is not mandatory. Place in the fridge until you intend to deep fry.

Heat your deep fryer to 170°C (338°F).

Cook the chicken until golden brown on the outside, approximately 10–12 minutes. Do not rush this process. Nobody wants to get salmonella. If you have a particularly thick piece of chicken, consider slicing it in half at the thickest part and checking to see whether it has any raw bits.

Remove your chicken from the deep fryer and allow it to cool on a dripping rack.

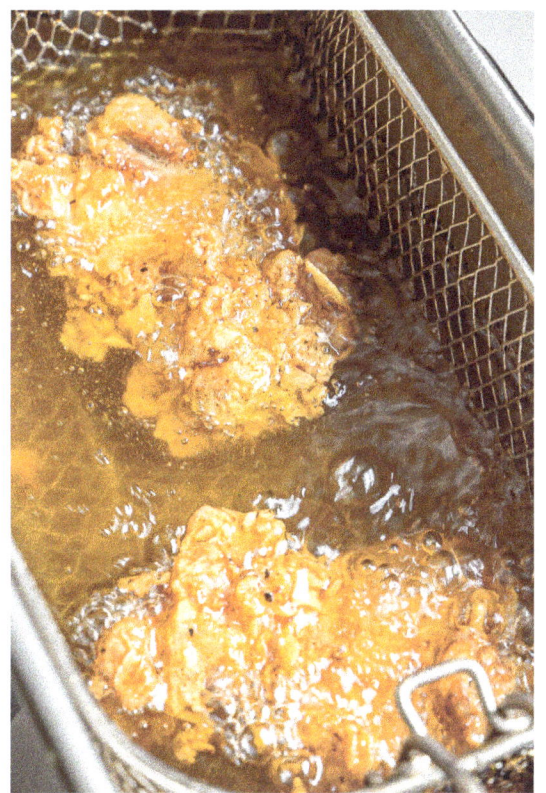
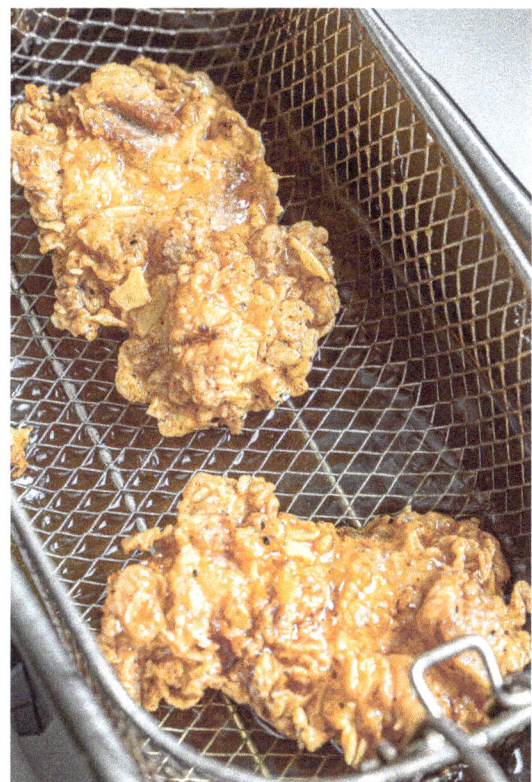

THE SANDWICH

1 brioche or milk bun

1 tbsp of chili jam

40 g of sliced red onion

1 slice of American hi melt cheese

Slice your red onion into 2–3 mm slivers.

Slice your brioche/milk bun in half.

Preheat your frying pan to a medium heat.

Place the inside of your cut buns on the grill, placing a small amount of pressure on them. Wait until they become soft and airy, and slightly brown on the inside. Remove and put aside for assembly.

By now your chicken should have dried, with most of the excess oil removed. Melt your cheese on the frying pan on a medium heat and remove with a nonstick spatula. Place the cheese on your chicken.

Assemble the burger—don't forget your chili jam!

Eat and enjoy.

THE MI-SO HUNGRY

It's very rare that I like to season a burger with anything other than salt (and sometimes pepper). As much as keeping it simple is smart, it's nice to change up your game here and there. I'm adverse to simply barbecue sauce basting my burgers. I want more than just sweet/smoky profiles if I'm going to bump up my flavor game. It reminds me of those over-sauced, often quite fatty, pork ribs you'd get from a pub that just tasted like a mouthful of $2 Homebrand barbecue sauce. For those watching at home, in Australia, Homebrand is our generic brand.

So, I went in search of different sauces I could baste my burgers in. I *love* Asian-style flavors cooked into burgers, so I wanted to find a way to give it a bit of a kick—umami and *oomph*—with a miso paste and sriracha hot sauce. But it would be rude of me to venture too far from the classic barbecue sauce basting that you often get. I was lucky enough to have a bottle of this *amazing* swineapple barbecue sauce from my local butcher, Tender Gourmet Butchery in Warringah Mall.

So, there I had it, a great little basting sauce that would work well with some thiccc patties. The rest just made sense to me: pork crackling for a crunch element, staying in tune with the *swine* part of swineapple. I searched for a great little jam or relish that would go hand in hand with the pork crackles, and I opted for a mango chutney for a bit of spice and sweetness, finishing it with some pickles (always) and a simple Truff hot sauce/mayonnaise combo. Safe to say, this isn't for the fainthearted. There's a plethora of overpowering and intense flavors here. But if you're looking for a flavor bomb, you're in luck.

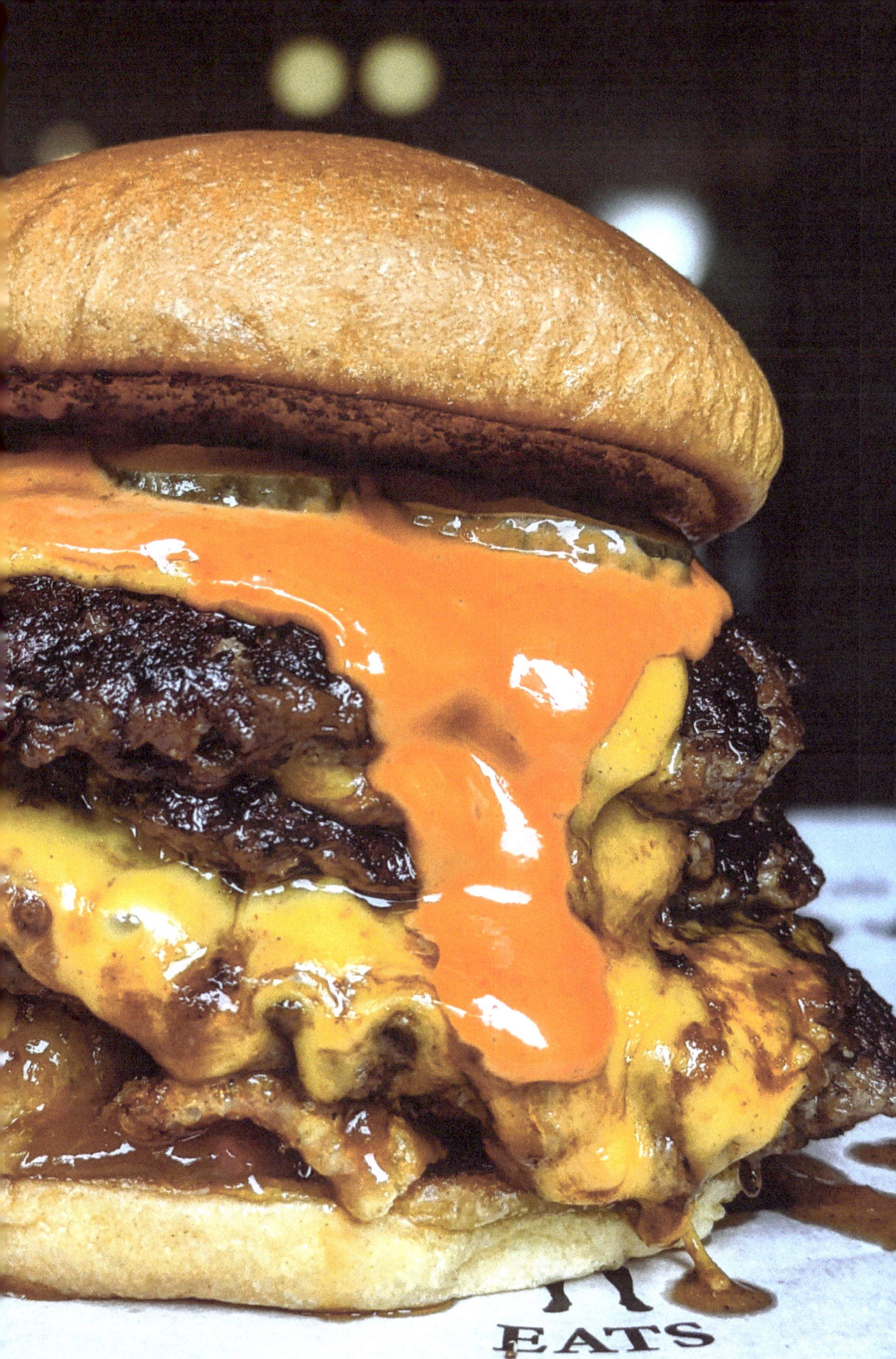

THE SAUCE

20 ml of Truff hot sauce (or a similar alternative)

30 ml of whole egg mayonnaise

In 2 small bowls, take your basting and sauce ingredients and stir them with a spoon until consistent and smooth.

THE BASTE

1 tsp of miso paste

1 tbsp of your favorite BBQ sauce

1 tbsp of sriracha hot sauce

THE BURGER

1–3 x 120 g balls of beef mince

1–3 slices of American hi melt cheese

1 brioche or milk bun

1 tbsp of mango chutney

½ cup of dried pork crackling (like the bar snack)

4–5 slices of dill pickle

Slice your brioche/milk bun in half.

Preheat your grill to a medium heat.

Place the inside of your cut buns on the grill, placing a small amount of pressure on them. Wait until they become soft and airy, and slightly brown on the inside. Remove and put aside for assembly.

Heat your grill up to a high temperature, wait until it's smoking hot, and place your patties on the grill one by one, leaving space between them to be flattened out.

Using your preferred smashing tool—you can either opt for a flat smash or an edged smash—press down your patties to just wider than your bun width. Apply your basting sauce to the uncooked side of the patty. Once the bottom side has caramelized, flip and allow for the basting sauce to cook into the patty. Leave this a little longer than you usually would, because you want the sauce to caramelize into the meat. Place your American cheese on the cooked side of the patty and wait to melt. Once melted, remove the patties from the grill and prepare to assemble your burger.

With the remaining ingredients, assemble your burger.

Eat and enjoy!

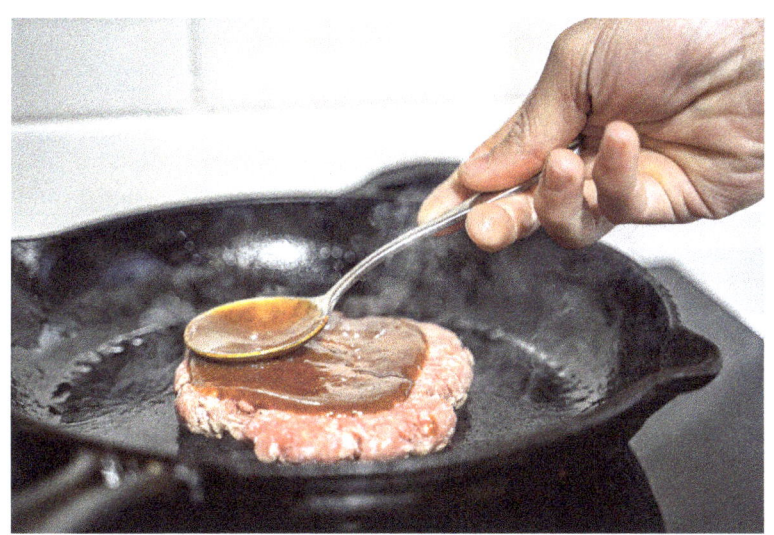

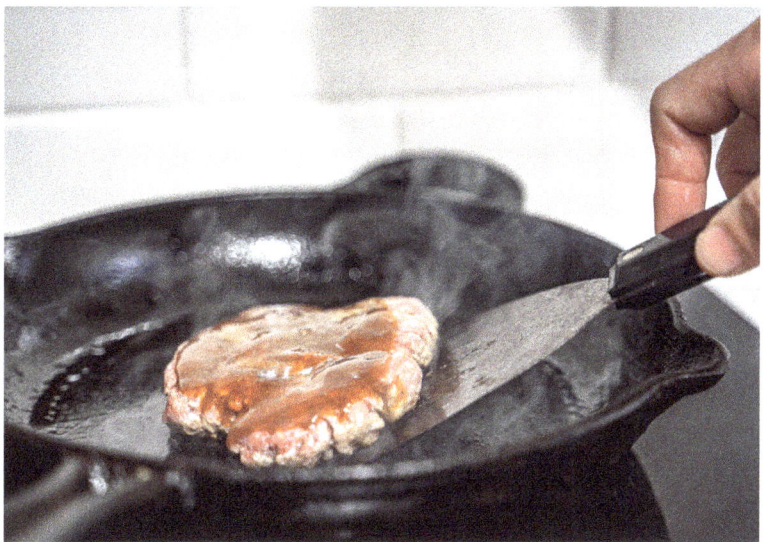

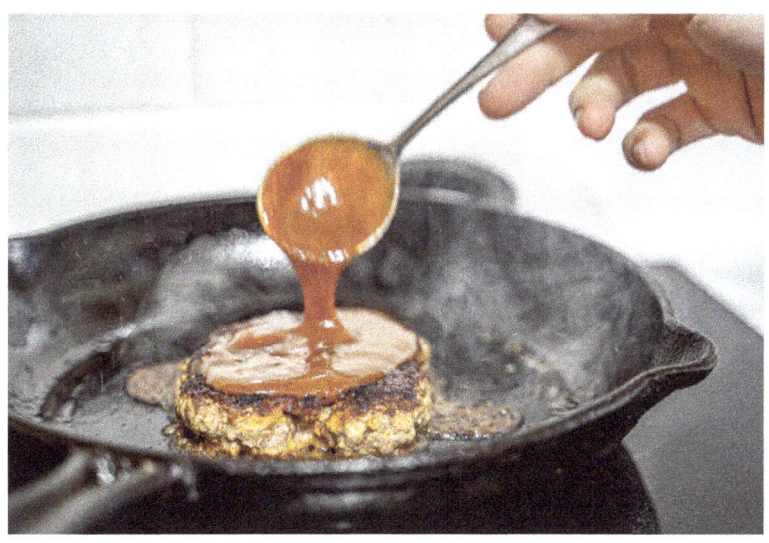

THE HUM DINGER BUM STINGER

Believe it or not, I was a glutton for punishment when it came to spicy food growing up. I can remember on many occasions wiping the sweat off my brow while I attempted to shovel down one of my Narni's famously hot curries. I was the type of guy who would bring his own bottle of hot sauce to events and put it on everything. I even managed to score a bottle of Flashbang hot sauce extract from a mate returning from the United States, which I couldn't help but put into my homemade chilies for an extra kick. The things I used to do make this burger seem like a cold, creamy Maccas McFlurry. But I had to stop after I pushed it too far, too many times. I attempted Australia's hottest pizza at Talotta's in Kurnell, and the aftermath was a nightmare I thought was never going to end.

So, here's one for you guys out there who just want to give yourself hell, without killing yourself. Pre-warning—the heat of this burger is completely up to you and your tolerance. If you believe you can take more heat, that's your decision, and you can increase it by adding hotter chilies. The beauty of this one is that it's customizable to you and what you like in a chili. I take no responsibility for you silly buggers. Sounds great, right?

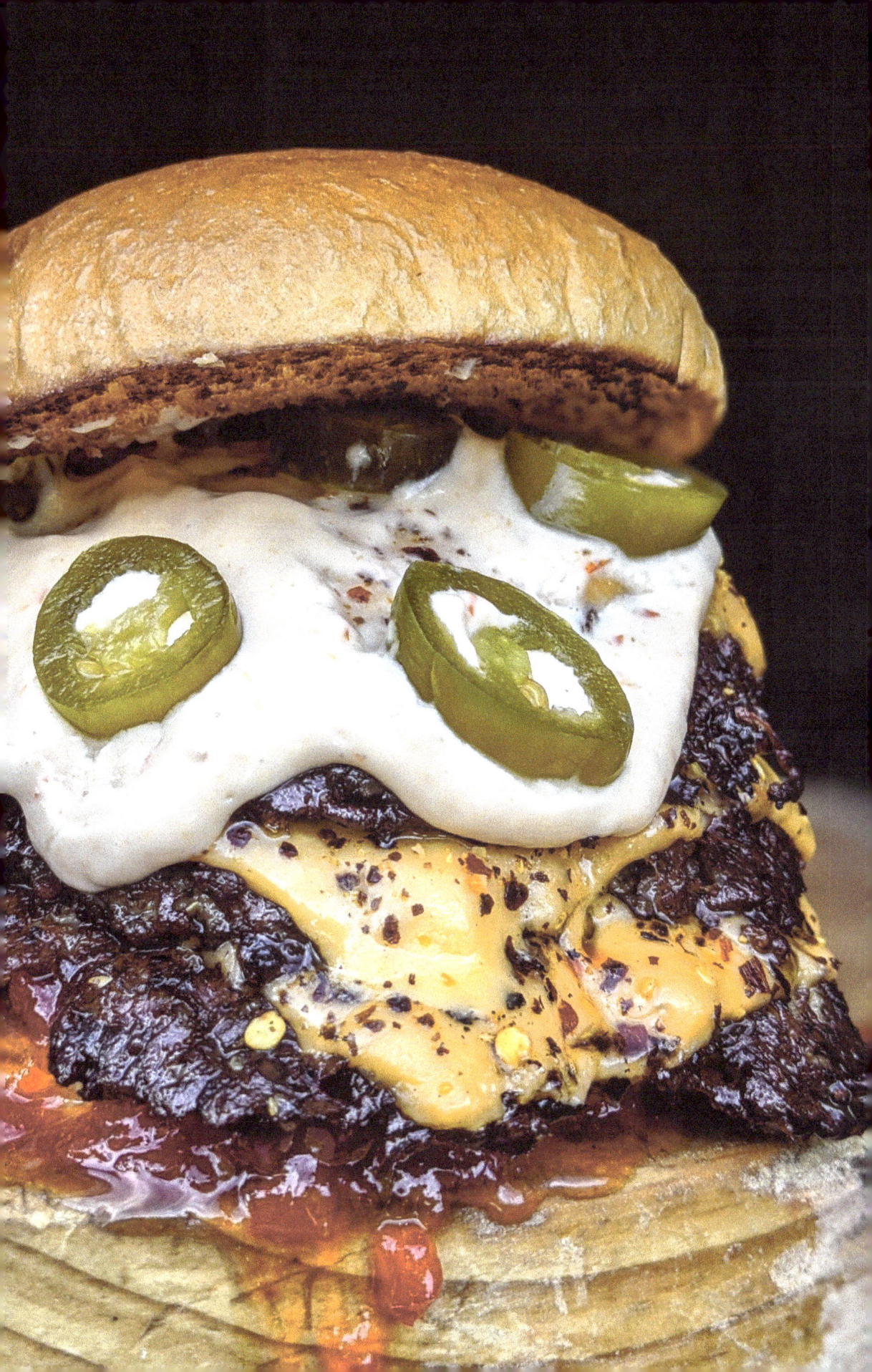

THE SAUCE

30 ml of whole egg mayonnaise

20 ml of your favorite hot sauce

In a small bowl, take the sauce ingredients and mix together until the mixture is consistent.

THE BURGER

1–3 x 100 g balls of beef mince

1–3 slices of American cheese (or jalapeño cheese if you can find it)

1–3 pinches of dried chili flakes (dealer's choice)

1–3 pinches of sea salt

4–6 slices of pickled jalapeños (or your choice of chili)

1 tbsp of chili jam

1 soft brioche or milk bun

Slice your brioche/milk bun in half.

Preheat your grill to a medium heat.

Place the inside of your cut buns on the grill, placing a small amount of pressure on them. Wait until they become soft and airy, and slightly brown on the inside. Remove and put aside for assembly.

Heat your grill up to a high temperature, wait until it's smoking hot, and place your patties on the grill one by one, leaving space between them to be flattened out.

Using your preferred smashing tool—you can either opt for a flat smash or an edged smash—press down your patties to just wider than your bun width. Season with a pinch of sea salt and your choice of dried chili. Once the bottom side of the patty has caramelized, flip and apply your American or jalapeño cheese. Wait until the cheese has melted, then remove from the grill for assembly.

Assemble the burger with your remaining ingredients.

Eat and enjoy!

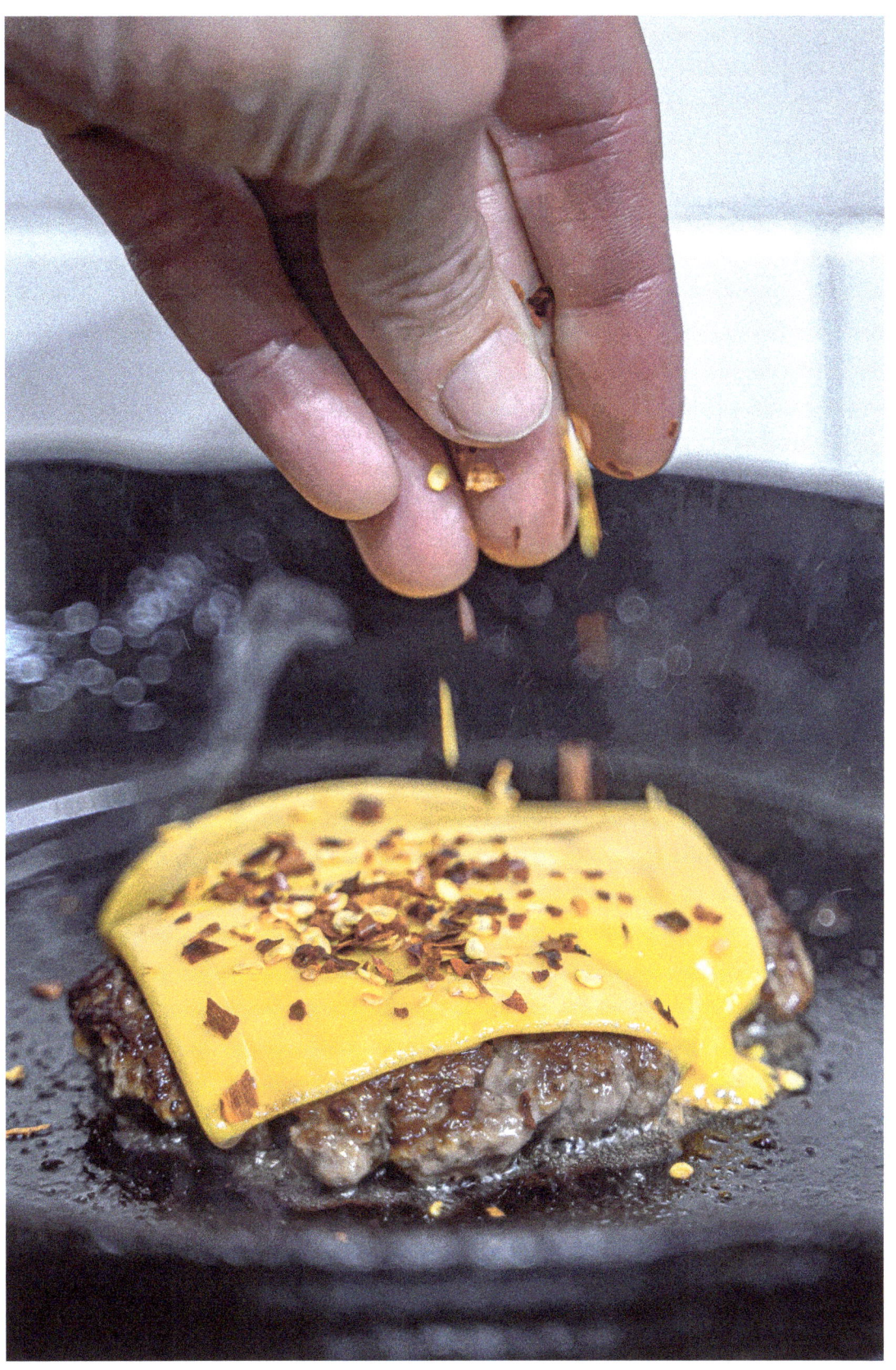

THE DOWN UNDAAAAH

If you hadn't noticed already, I'm painfully Australian. I'm the kind of guy who goes to the "footy" for a few "schooeys" and may even dabble in a "shoey." I call my best mates, whose names are Damon and Simon, "Damo and Simo." I pronounce Australia with a simple "straya." I'll shorten almost any word to the point of complete confusion for other people. Most people call it a U-turn, and most Aussies call it a U-ey. I call it a "yuzza." I'll cook my lamb on the barby, throw back a few cans, and chuck a footy with my mates. I'll have a slap on the pokies, have a punt on the trots, and drink a pot.

Aussie culture is bloody awesome. And we have a burger that is so painfully Aussie, it also calls a U-turn a yuzza and its mates Damo and Simo: the Australian works burger. You'd be hard-pressed to not find at least one shop in each suburb across most of Australia that doesn't sell a works burger. It's nostalgic for most Aussies, and quite literally the lifeblood of a lot of tradies. It has a long list of ingredients that will make you scratch your noggin', but it's cheap as chips to make and simple as a Queenslander (or Kweenlander) to put together.

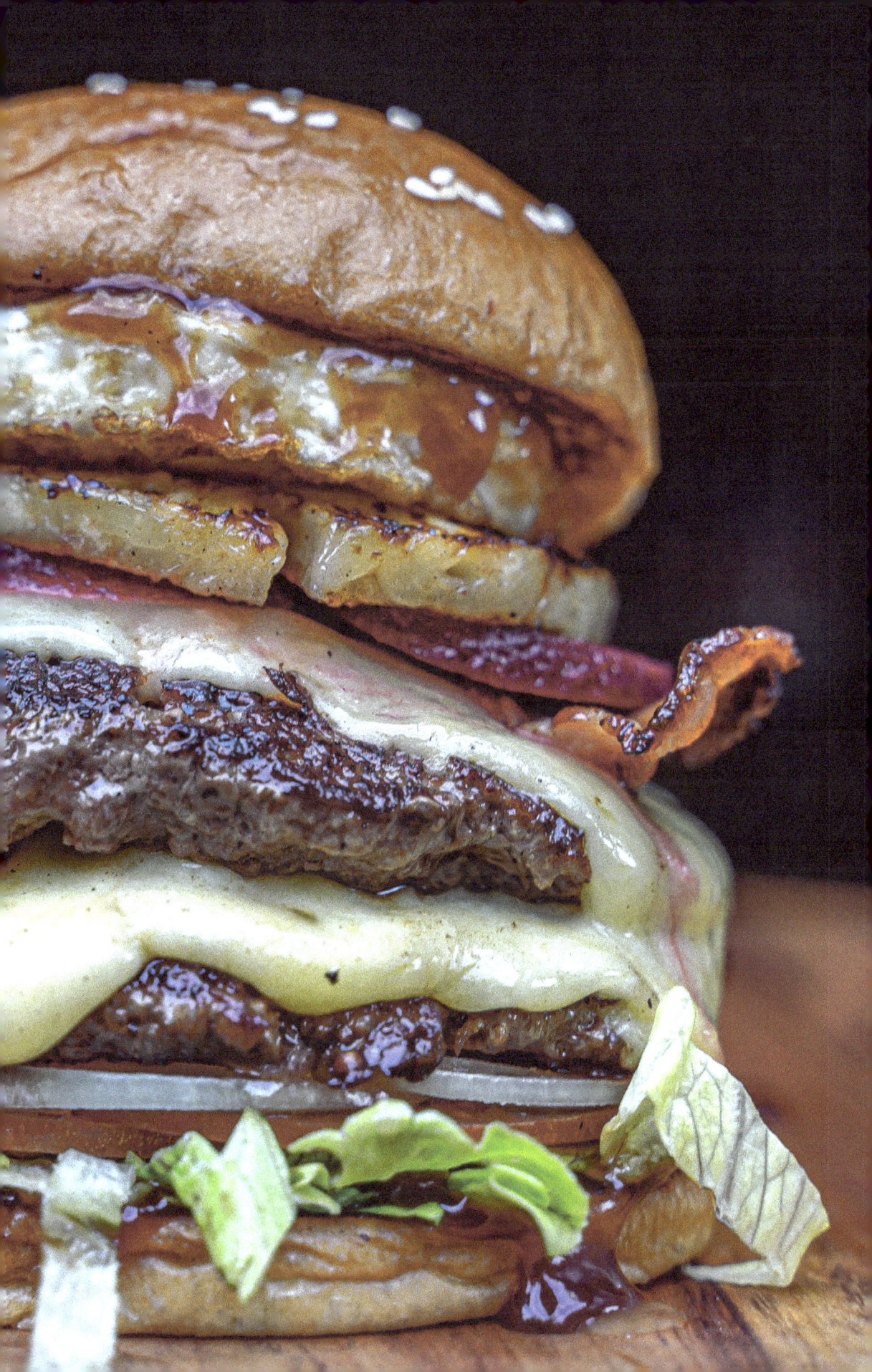

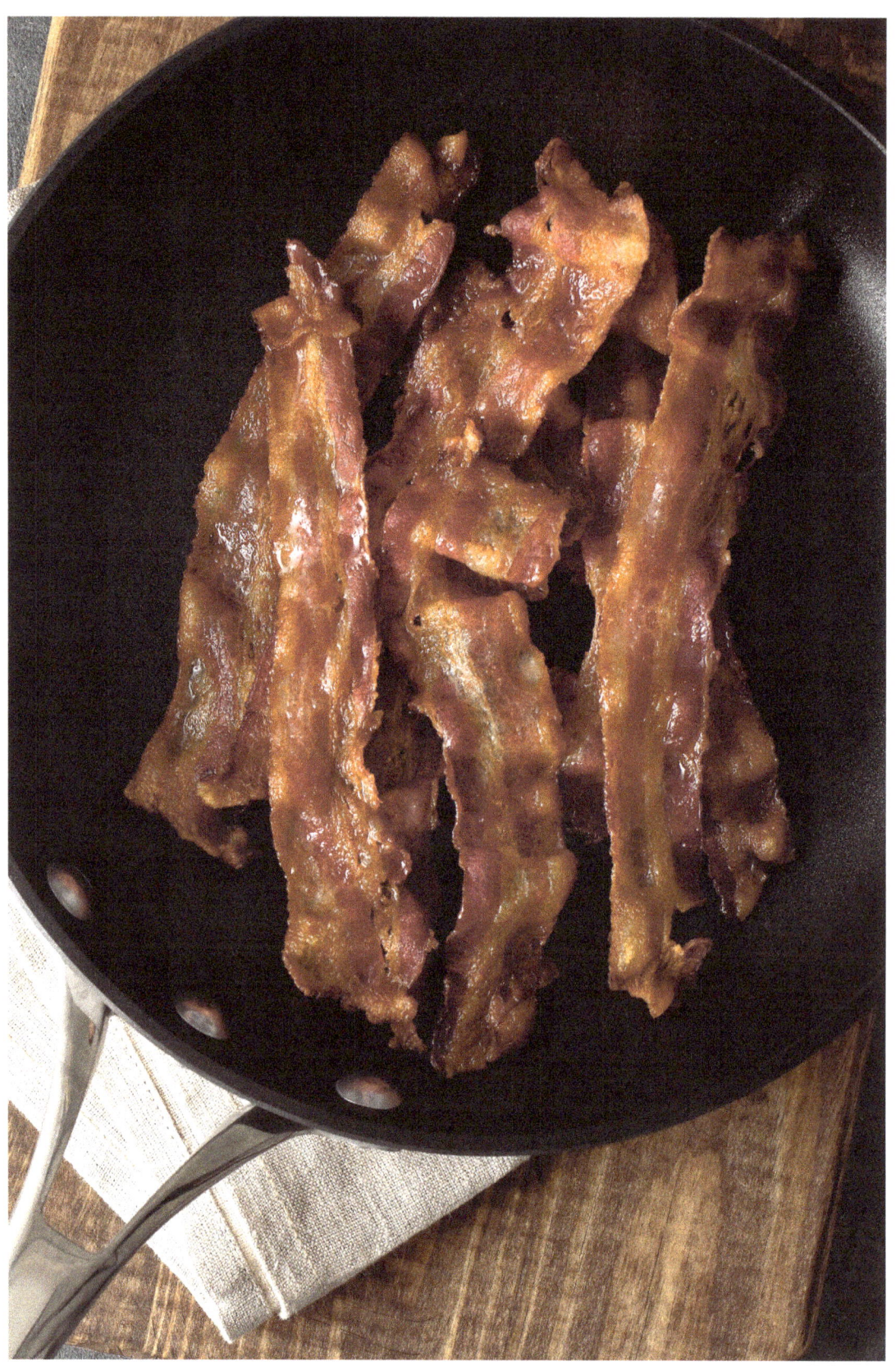

THE BURGER

¼ cup of shredded iceberg lettuce

2 rings of canned pineapple slices

3 slices of canned beetroot

1 extra-large egg

1 small brown onion

1–3 x 100g balls of beef mince

1–3 slices of cheddar

2 pieces of streaky bacon

30 ml of barbecue sauce

1 sesame seed roll

Slice your sesame seed roll in half.

Slice your onion into thin rings, placing 2–3 aside for the burger.

Preheat your grill to a medium heat.

Place the inside of your cut buns on the grill, placing a small amount of pressure on them. Wait until they become soft and airy, and slightly brown on the inside. Remove and put aside for assembly.

Heat your grill up to a high temperature, wait until it's smoking hot, and place your patties on the grill one by one, leaving space between them to be flattened out. Place your bacon on the other side of the hot grill.

Using your preferred smashing tool—you can either opt for a flat smash or an edged smash—press down your patties to just wider than your bun width. Season with a pinch of sea salt. Once the bottom side of the patty has caramelized, flip and apply your cheddar cheese. Wait until the cheese has melted, then remove the patties from the grill for assembly.

Crack your egg onto the grill where the leftover bacon fat is and cook to your preference (I like sunny side up).

Assemble your burger using all ingredients.

Eat and enjoy!

THE FINAL CHAPTER

It has been quite a ride writing this book. I feel so privileged to have had the capacity to do this and that you have all been along for the journey. I want to leave you with one last anecdote, and I hope it brings you as much joy as it does to me.

Food is more than a vehicle for us to remember moments in our lives; it also connects us to the *people* in our lives. I'm so lucky to be able to carry the memories of people through our shared food experiences.

My incredible mother, Kerrie, nurtured me at a very young age and taught me that I could be the cook as a husband. She took the time to let me cook with her. A young Jesse would stand on a stool, just tall enough to see over the kitchen counter, and help Mum cook, although, I'm sure I was more of a hindrance. She was patient and gave me the time to understand things, rather than just trying to hurry me through it. To this day, we still cook together and get excited to tell each other about amazing recipes we've tried.

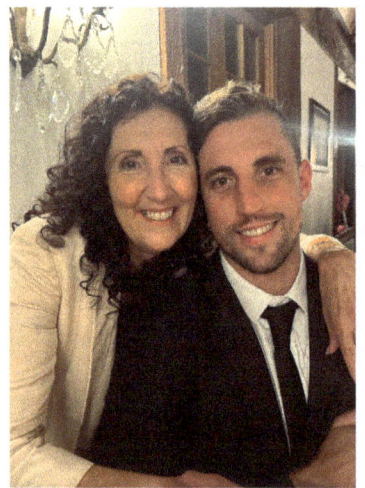

My hardworking dad, Mark, taught me the importance of traditions behind food: how it's important to conduct yourself at the dinner table, how to be a polite host, and to make sure everyone always has a drink in their hand. He taught me about keeping Sundays for relaxing and did so by frying up whatever leftovers there were from the night before as "bubble and squeak." He'd make me peanut butter toast with lashings of butter after my weekend sport and challenge me on my thoughts about my performance.

My late nanna, Flo, taught me about the importance of bringing together family with food. It wasn't a Christmas dinner without her amazing pork crackling, and she'd always make a mouthwatering roast with all the trimmings. On our family trips to Forster, lunch was filled with laughter and stories of the day as Nanna worked away in the kitchen, cooking rissoles and assembling sandwiches for us all.

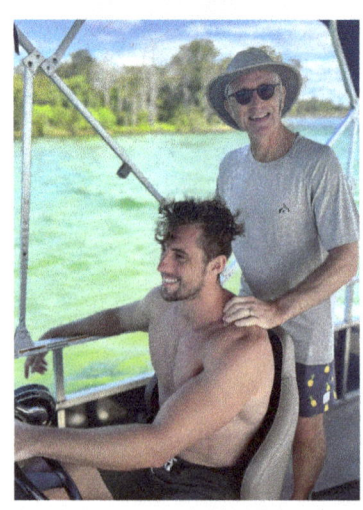

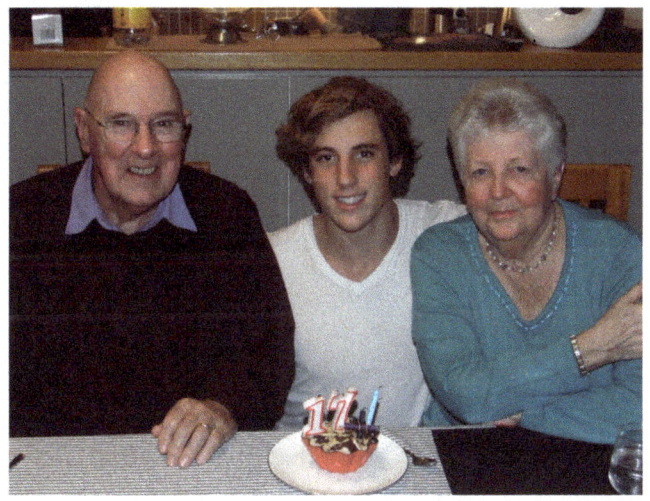
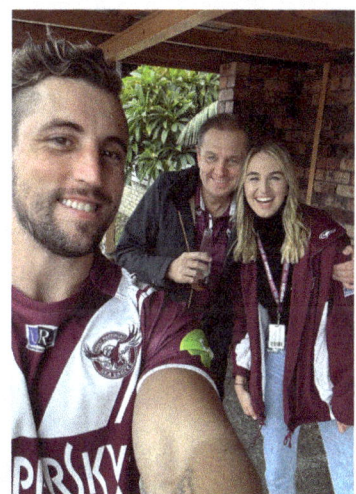

My father-in-law, Paul, and my late grandad, Walter, taught me the importance of taking the time to have a drink with someone. It doesn't matter what's going on in the world; sometimes you need to stop and give people your undivided attention. It took me a while to realize just how powerful it can be.

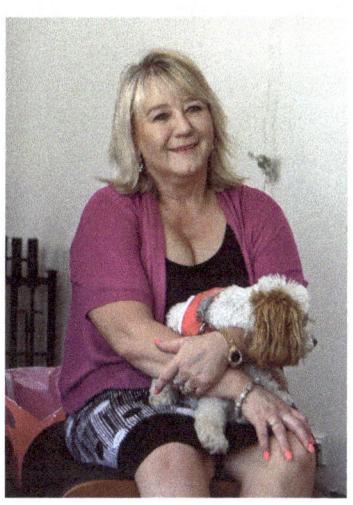

My late mother-in-law, Anna, taught me that food is a love language. She had this unforgettable knack for knowing exactly what people liked, and you'd be damn sure she'd always have it for you when you were visiting. For my brother-in-law, Tom, she'd always make sure there was Bundy rum in the fridge, for me, kombucha. She knew that I loved her chicken schnitzels and would often make them for me, just to see my elated reaction. She would talk excitedly to me about butchers and cooking utensils she had found, knowing that I loved talking about them. She showed me just how special you can make someone feel by making an effort to know what they like.

Food is so much more than just something we eat. It's the memories of events and people it carves into our minds. It's a reminder of the good times, and sometimes the bad.

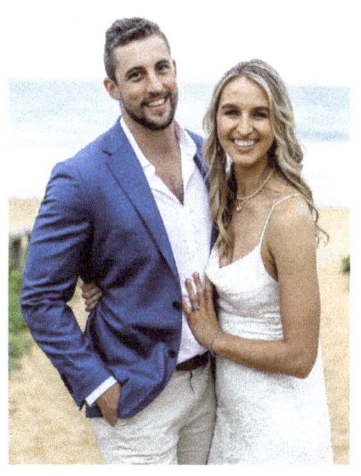

I hope I've inspired you to look at food in a completely new way and cherish it like I do. When you make these burgers, remember, they can be more than just food. They can mark pivotal moments in your memory, and your life.

SPECIAL MENTIONS

Now for some special mentions ...

I couldn't very well wrap up *The Foodcoma Cookbook* without paying homage to some of the most inspiring and influential burgers—and their creators—from my burger journey. Many of these creations forever changed the way I think about food.

From the epically imaginative to the downright delicious, each and every mention holds a special place in my heart and history. I hope they inspire you as much as they did me.

Let the final feast begin!

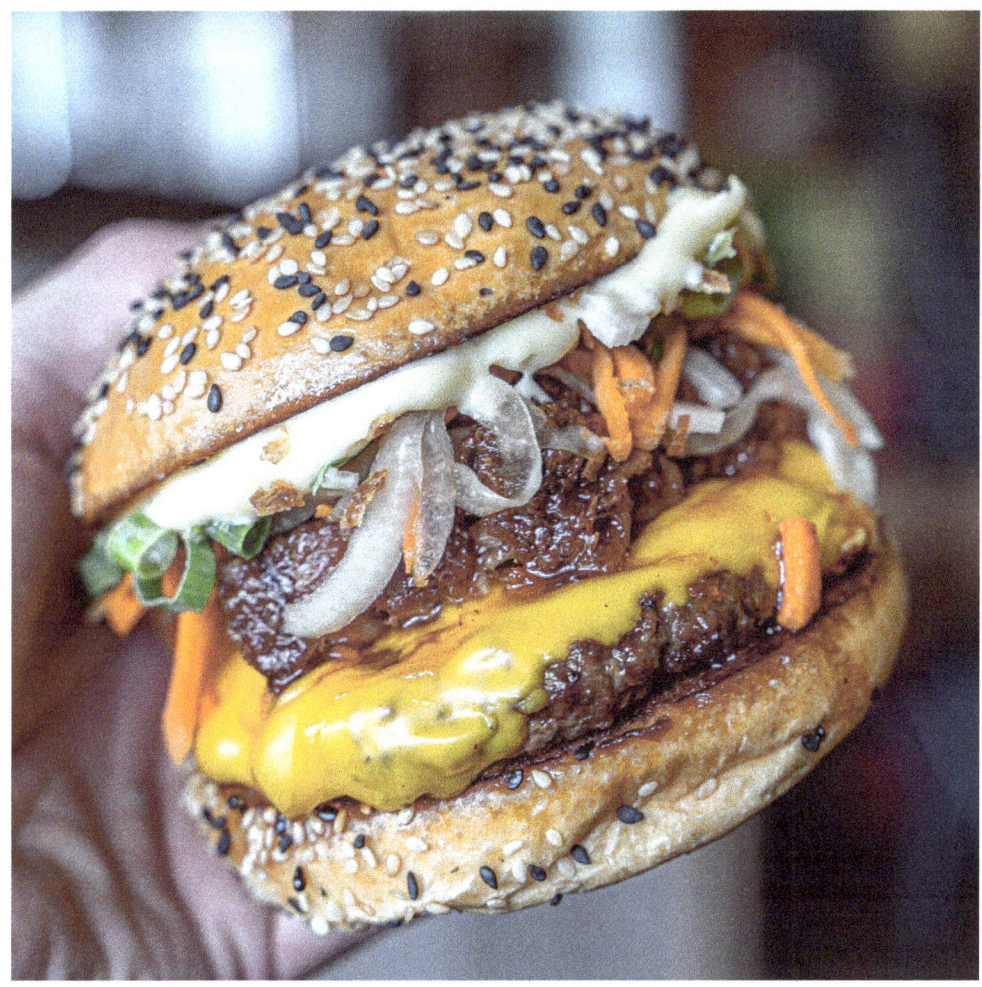

THE MR MIYAGI
BY TWO HUNGRY BEARS

If there's one burger that has changed the way I think about food, it's the "Mr Miyagi" from Two Hungry Bears in Narrabeen, NSW. Many years ago, I met the owner of a cafe in Brookvale. His name was Clinton and after connecting the dots, we realized that we both had grown up in the same suburb, Terrey Hills. As it turned out, we had many mutual friends and knew several of each other's family members.

When I was starting my burger journey, his quaint shop in Brookvale was a regular pit stop for me, as he would bring out a new and delicious burger every week. It was a tiny cafe, located up a long and steep driveway, that served (almost) exclusively the offices situated above and anyone daring enough to park below and hike up to his shop. We had a simple relationship: he would make me a mouthwatering burger, and I would snap a couple of pictures that he could use on social media.

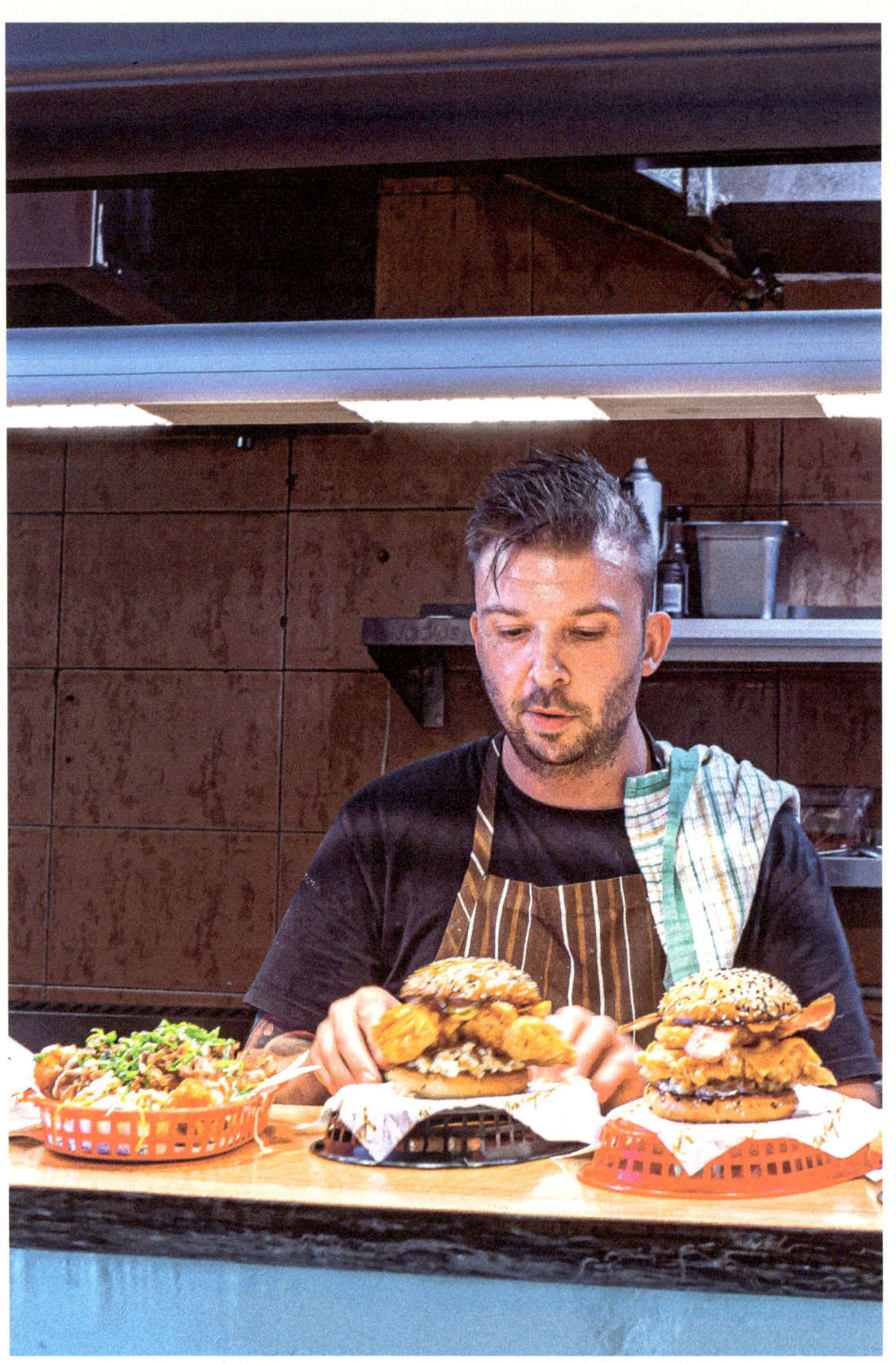

It wasn't long before we developed a friendship. I recall telling stories about our lives and meeting his toddler, Indie. I even did a celebrity shift at the shop. Eventually, we started working together. I took over his social media page and started regularly photographing his food, and it wasn't long before things took off. One year, he invited me to his work Christmas party, and Mr Miyagi was born.

During the event, we attended a beautiful restaurant in the heart of Sydney. There, we sat down, drank a couple beers, and made our way through an elegant menu of small dishes. One dish in particular stood out: sweet and sour, deep fried pork hock. Quite a mouthful, aye? We all took one cube each of this crunchy piece of meat candy. Slowly, we all started to eat. Our eyes lit up as the pork broke up into phenomenal strings of flavor, each chew giving a satisfying, crispy texture. We had found nirvana. We quickly began to discuss how the dish could be put into a burger. When it comes to conversations that take place after a couple of beers, you expect them to be quickly forgotten, like that one time you promised your mates you'd all go skydiving next weekend. But it was different this time.

The following Monday, I received a text from Clinton: "I think we've got a unicorn here" (unicorn was a term used by burger enthusiasts in Sydney for the best burger they'd ever had). I hurried over to his shop in Brookvale, sprinted up the driveway, and arrived sweating and breathing heavily. As Clinton cooked the burger, I listened to Zac, the front-of-house, rave on about this unicorn I would soon experience for myself. Finally, the burger came out, and I knew I was in for something special.

Built on a soft, pillow-like milk bun, the Mr Miyagi became my favorite burger in Sydney. It consisted of a patty that had been licked by flames and charred beautifully by the grill. The interior of the patty had a slight hue of pink; the juices slowly oozed out to the exterior, and a mouthful of umami, salt, and a slight bitterness rounded it out. Then there was a simple slice of American hi melt cheese, hugging the meat with tight arms, melted to provide a touch of gooeyness and saltiness. Next up was the glorious pork hock. I don't know the specifics of what he did to it, but it was just as I remembered it from the restaurant in Sydney: punching with sweet, sour, and umami flavors, coming together with a delightful crispiness, which then broke down to a moreish, stringy texture. A layer of sweet-pickled vegetables provided a much-needed freshness and acidity, and the burger was finished with a small pinch of fried onion, fresh shallots for a kick, and an earthy, creamy sesame mayonnaise.

I moaned my way through my first few bites. I couldn't contain the animalistic pleasure I felt eating that burger. In a few moments, which consisted of a flurry of biting, moaning, slurping, and smiling, the burger was gone. It felt like nothing I'd ever experienced before. I'm sure you'd be glad to know, Clinton has made a name for himself now. We still work together, and I have no doubt we will be forever bound by this burger.

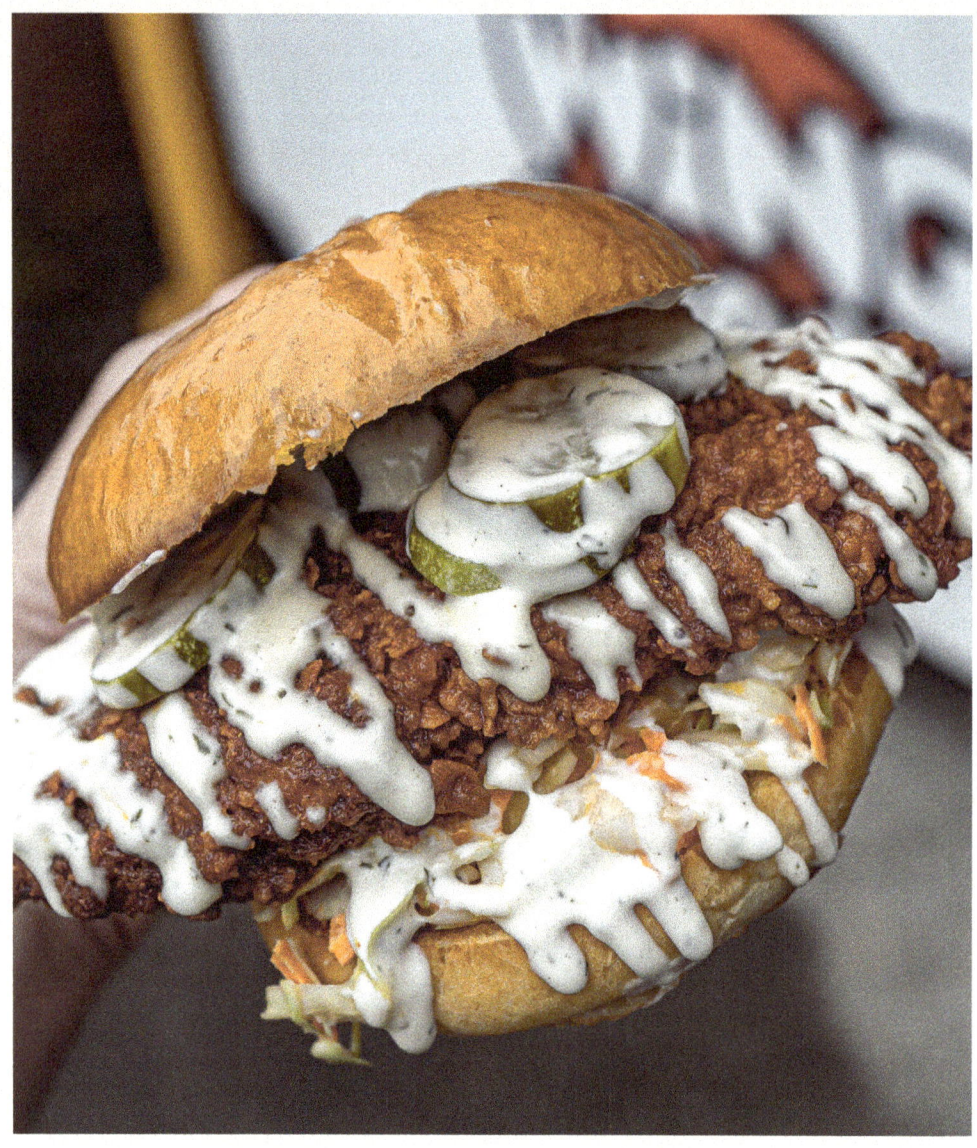

THE NASHVILLE HOT BURGER
WING SHACK

Years before Nashville fried chicken was a big thing in Sydney, I was invited to try out Wing Shack in Kings Park. It was nearly an hour's drive from my Insular Peninsula (what they call the Northern Beaches), but I wasn't one to turn down some delicious fried chicken. Arriving in Kings Park, I didn't know what to expect from a restaurant there. The area is littered with construction companies, mechanics, car dealerships, and plenty of industrial land. The shop was in a line of four other shops, a very unassuming store without any of the pizazz of a restaurant. All this language might seem negative to you, but, to me, this is *exactly* what made it so special. I had found a truly undiscovered gem.

I met with the owners, Joel and Rob, a yin and yang team, almost polar opposites. But they had two things in common: their love affair with fried chicken and their passion for delivering a phenomenal product. I sat outside with my then girlfriend (now wife), Kira, and waited patiently for our fried chicken to arrive. It came out and to my absolute surprise, it was glowing red, with a grainy layer on top of the mountainous crispy and craggy bits of southern fried coating. With no clue what Nashville fried chicken was, I bit into it and immediately had a coughing fit. I had breathed in the spicy Nashville dusting, without knowing it had cayenne pepper and chili powder in it. I laughed and regrouped, determined to show this radioactive chicken who was the man—and recover some man points in front of my wife to be.

What came next was an experience that has stayed with me ever since and made me love Nashville fried chicken. The southern fried coating gave way with a resounding CRUNCH as I took my bite, the crispy exterior mixing with the sweet, salty, smoky, and spicy cayenne butter (the red stuff). The chicken inside was unbelievably succulent, juicy, and bursting with flavor. Each bite brought together an array of textures, flavors, and spiciness. After mowing down my first tender, I noticed that the cayenne was catching up to me, and I quickly sank a couple sips of Coke Zero to keep the heat beast at bay.

Then it was time to face a monster of a burger: the Nashville Hot Burger. It was layered with delicate lines of cool ranch, a creamy coleslaw, huge thick dill pickles, and a large white bun. I knew this was going to be my favorite, so I rushed to dibs it. The creamy coleslaw, cool ranch, and white bun provided the perfect heat resistant team, while allowing enough heat to come through to keep me salivating and alert.

I quickly fell in love with the burger and started bringing as many friends as I could to the spot. It wasn't long before I began blasting on my social media about this new product that was in Sydney. I would visit regularly, bringing along other food bloggers from all walks of life, excitedly explaining to them the intricacies of Nashville chicken. It didn't take long for Nashville fried chicken to become quite popular in Sydney, and I've been lucky enough to try large quantities of it. However, you always remember your first experience, and mine was at Wing Shack. It still remains my favorite Nashville fried chicken in Sydney.

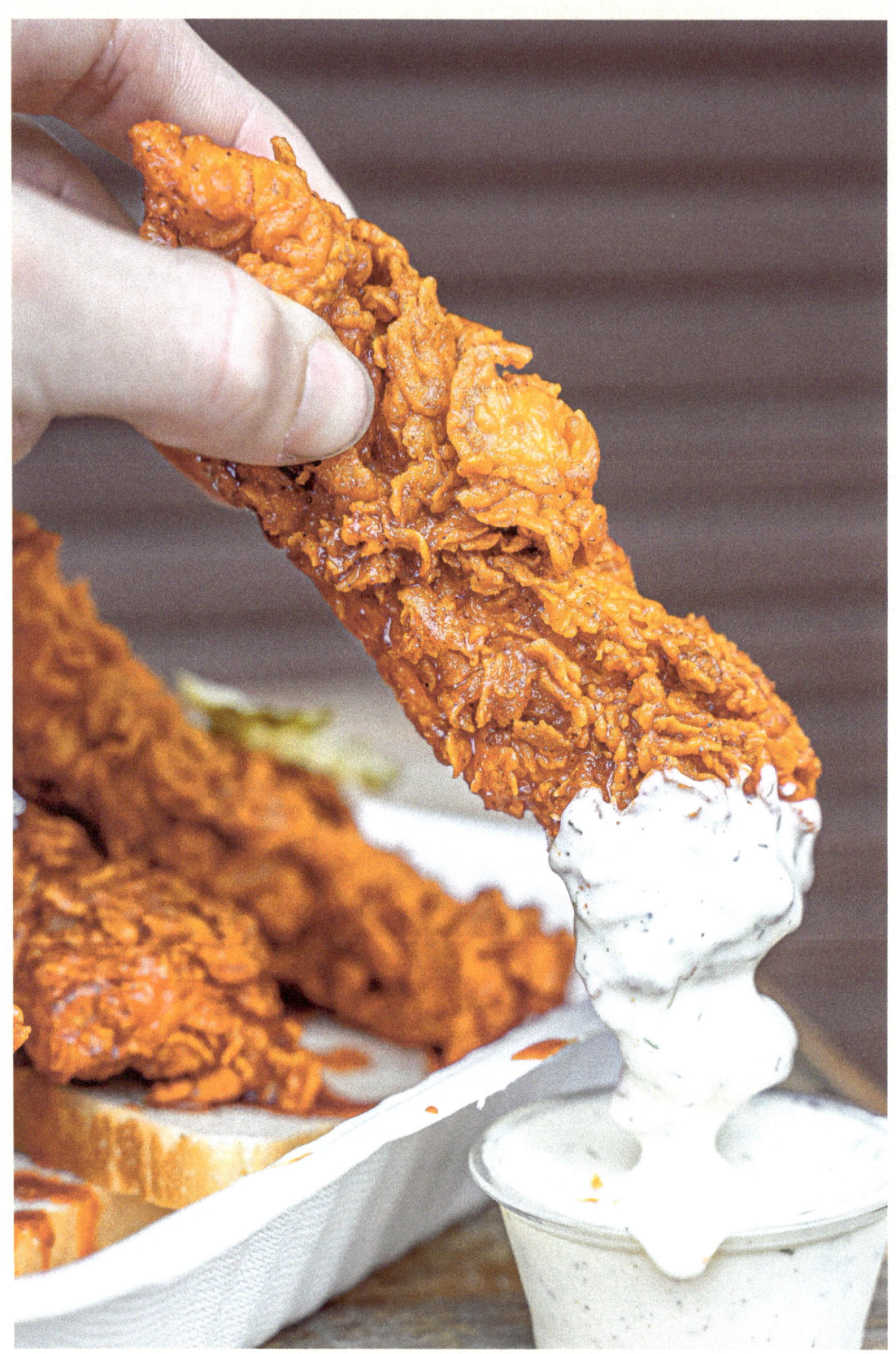

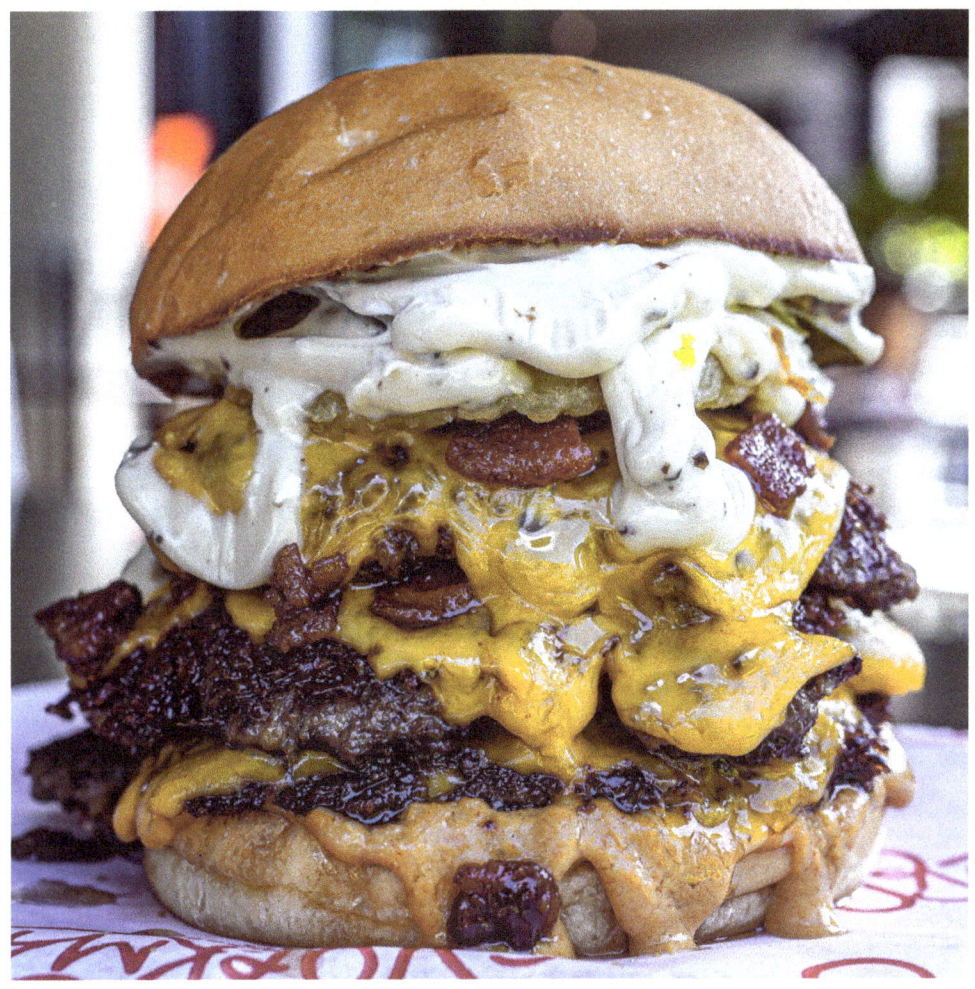

THE FOOD COMA HACK
STOCKMANS BBD DEE WHY

I'm sure there aren't many people in the world who can say they've had a burger hack named after them. I feel pretty chuffed that I'm one of a select few! The story of Stockmans starts well before I was obsessed with growing a burger Instagram. Believe it or not, it was one of the first places I took my wife in the early days of our relationship. We were freshly dating and in classic Jesse form, I took her on a beach date. After a couple hours talking and swimming at the beach, we wanted to continue hanging out. Considering you could have heard both our stomachs grumbling from a mile away, lunch was on the cards. Now, at the time, I was unbelievably neurotic about my diet. I was fasting strict hours, eating minimal calories, and exercising ten times a week. It exhausts me just thinking about it. Why did I think that was healthy? I thought it would be fun to visit a burger shop near the beach, so I broke my "healthy" habit for the day.

We both ordered burgers, and I got something called "The Maverick" because I thought it sounded cool. After sitting and playing Uno together at the table—they had cards there to keep people entertained—our food finally arrived, and we both tucked in without a word being said. I wasn't sure if it was the hunger speaking or the fact that I was infatuated with this girl, but that burger tasted pretty damn good.

Fast forward a couple years, and I returned to Stockmans, this time for content for my Instagram. A four-patty burger is likely to catch the attention of anyone, and it didn't take long for one of the owners, Corey, to come out and ask if I was "that Food Coma guy." I laughed because my order had given it away. We chatted for a few minutes, and Corey invited me to the opening of their new shop around the corner, which I attended.

It didn't take long for me to grow close with Corey and Bill, the owners of Stockmans. I would come in regularly and take photos and videos for them, and we would tell stories and talk about their product. We came up with weird and wacky burger specials together, and I soon realized I was obsessed with their caramelized bacon. One day, I asked for the Maverick, a burger that was special to me, but this time I wanted it as a triple, with caramelized bacon on every layer. It was a BIG burger, and also a BIG ask, but they obliged and pulled together an absolute masterpiece. Every angle of this burger was mouthwatering: layers of cheese, caramelized bacon, juicy beef, onion rings, pickles, truffle mayonnaise, a soft milk bun, and their signature Stockmans sauce. I dribbled a bit just writing this. Every photo I took was amazing, and the Maverick just popped with color and sharpness. I bit into the burger, and it was exactly what I wanted: a rich, sweet, and over-the-top combination of flavors, the caramelized bacon providing little morsels of crunch and sweetness to every layer. The photo went absolutely bananas on Instagram. It kept being posted and reposted by many pages that followed me. I was blown away. I kept ordering it every time I went in, and it wasn't long before they added it to their menu as "The Food Coma Hack," which is flattering for a guy who just took some pictures.

You'll be glad to know Stockmans is doing great. They serve a huge menu of drinks, crazy desserts, beers, fries, burgers, and more. Corey even visited me when I was out of work during the COVID pandemic, popping up in a food trailer and letting me flip burgers myself. I will never forget that. The boys have been very kind to me over the years, and I'll always support them in whatever ventures they undertake.

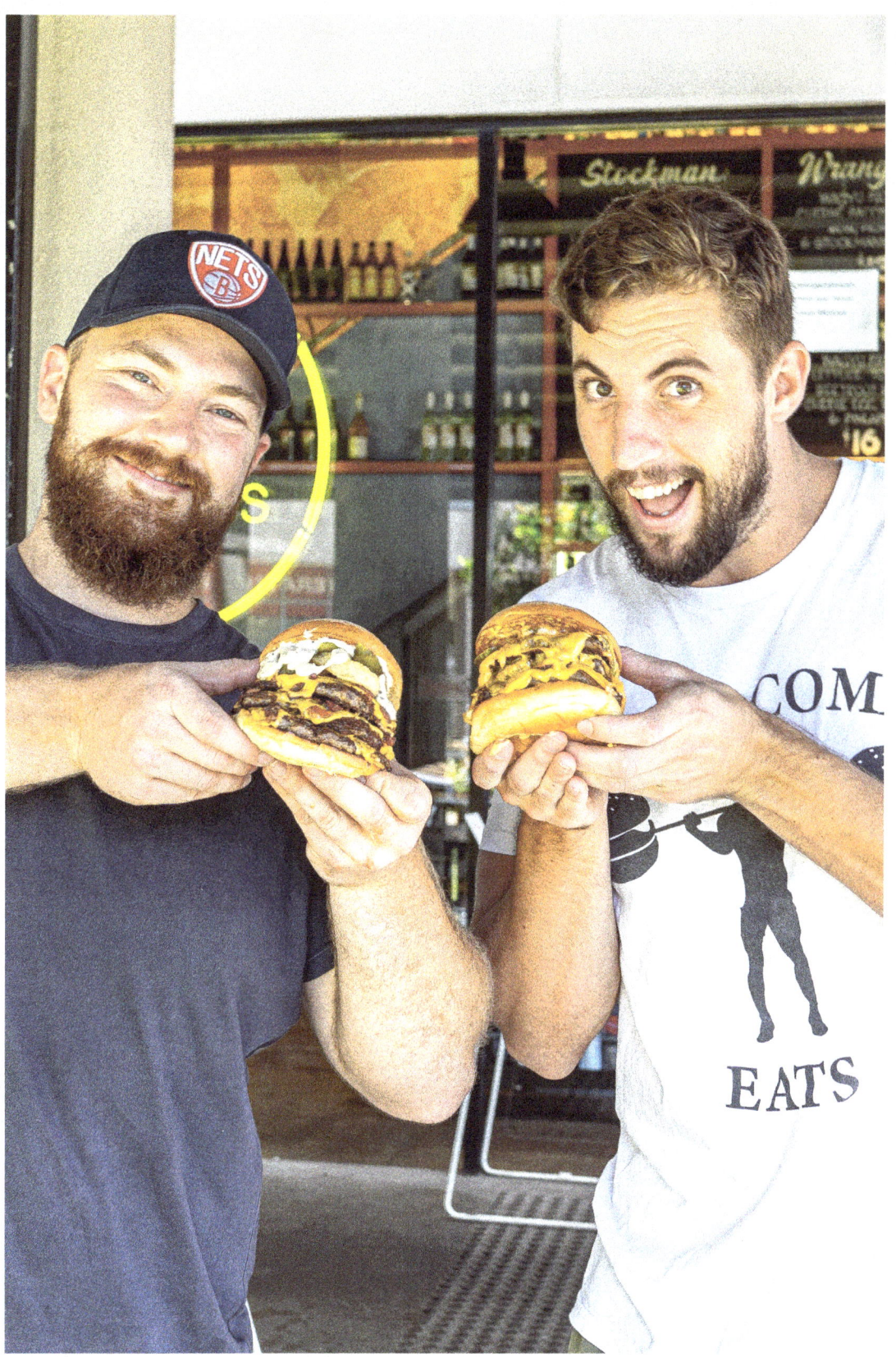

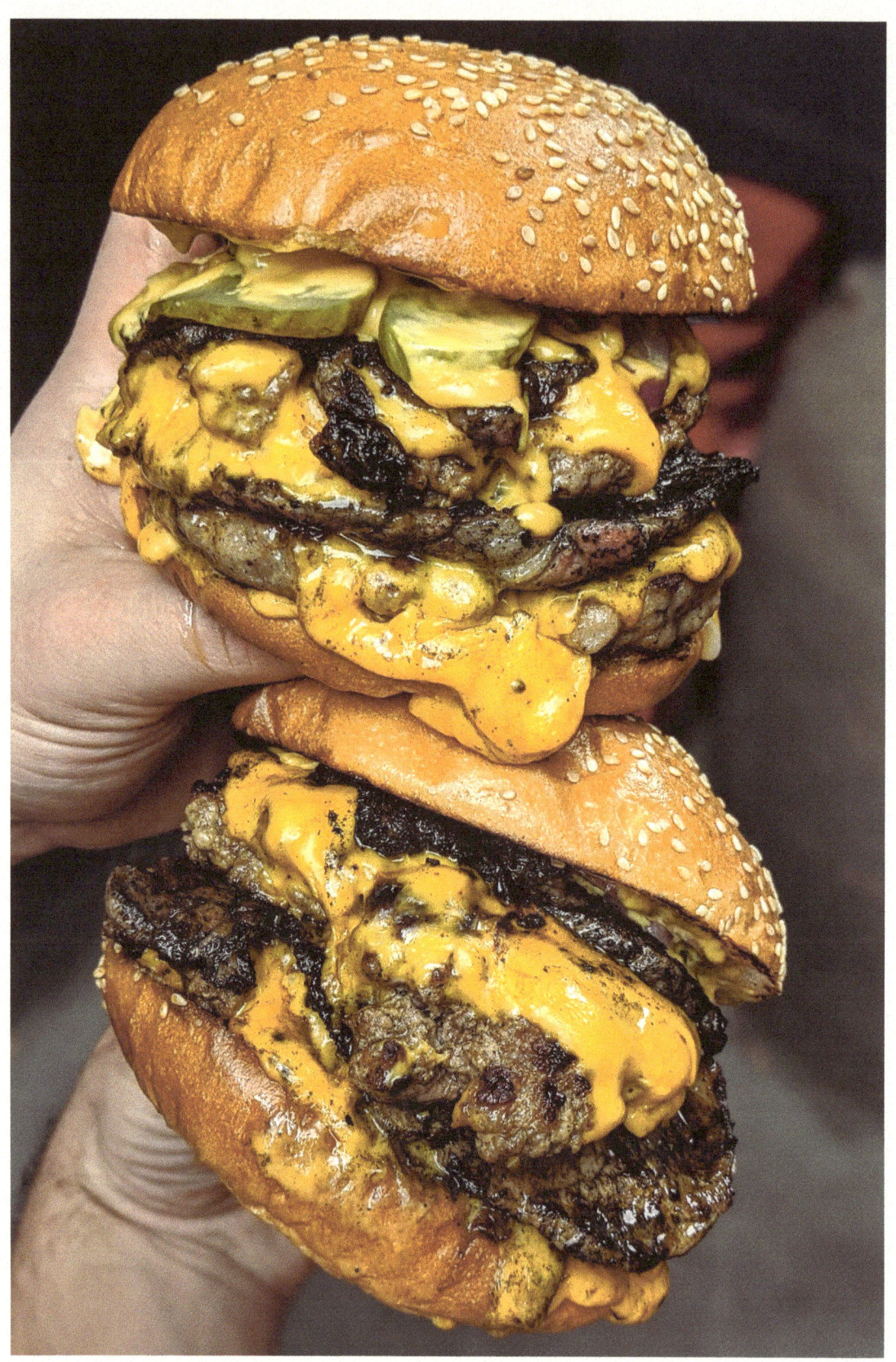

THE FOOD COMA BURGER

TENDER GOURMET BUTCHERY WARRINGAH MALL

I swear I'm not just here to mention burgers that are named after me, but I'd be remiss to not mention them in a book I'm writing...

Tender Gourmet Butchery (TGB)—I have unending respect for the guys here. Our story starts a bit on the crazy side, all thanks to my own stupidity.

A few years back, In-N-Out was doing a pop-up in Sydney. This was a big deal for Sydneysiders, as not many US fast food burger joints have come to Australia. I found out about the pop-up the morning of and immediately called my foodie bestie, Scott (the Wolf of Eat Street). He then chucked a sickie for work, and we rushed over to line up for In-N-Out in Surry Hills. As it turned out, we weren't the only people who had that idea. We were entrenched in a huge line that wrapped and snaked its way through the backstreets of Sydney. After an hour and a half of waiting, we finally walked through the doors, eagerly ordering our burgers, doing our Instagram thing, and getting out of there.

Scotty and I had scheduled to meet with the TGB guys at 2 p.m., and we left the city at 1 p.m., cutting it pretty close. After a rushed morning, we finally arrived in Brookvale via bus. I then scrolled through my messages to find out the location for the shop. My heart sank. I pressed "Get Directions" on Google Maps, and it told me the shop was in HORNSBY—forty minutes away. I was heartbroken. I felt so irresponsible for getting it wrong. I was unsure why I had Warringah Mall in my mind when planning out the day. I messaged them, apologizing profusely, saying that I'd be forty minutes late. I jumped in my car and did the drive to Hornsby, kicking myself the entire way for being so stupid.

I arrived and sprinted through the shopping center, frantically trying to find the butcher, not wanting to waste any more time. I finally arrived at the butcher and asked them if Adam was in. I was puzzled when they replied that he was at another store that day. I finally looked back at my messages, read the fine print, and realized that I was correct the first time. They asked me to come to Warringah Mall in Brookvale. I was defeated. What a farce! I summoned the courage to tell them what had happened and traveled back to Brookvale with my tail between my legs. The journey was complete.

I never made the same mistake again, and it wasn't long before Chris, the young butcher turned business owner, and I started talking about all things food. We would chat about our favorite rugby teams, talk about other burger restaurants, and brainstorm about food. He also showed me their equipment and the behind-the-scenes of their dry aging room. The best part—he always wanted to feed me his new burger creations.

One day, he said he wanted to put a thin slice of delicious, dry aged beef on a burger for me to try. I watched in anticipation as he took a house-ground 100 percent brisket patty and smashed it on the grill, creating

SPECIAL MENTIONS 145

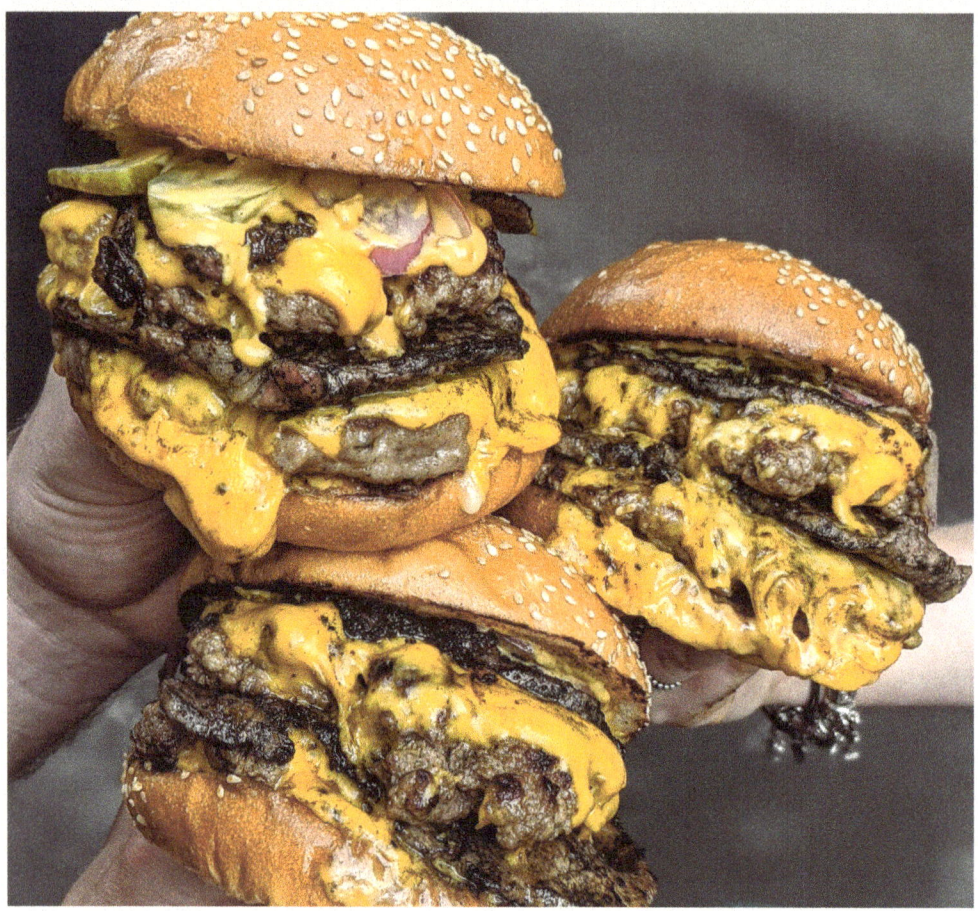

a beautiful crust of caramelization. He then took a beautifully marbled piece of dry aged beef, lightly coated it with a rub, and gave it a quick zap on the grill next to the cooking patty. He put it all together with an in-house burger sauce, pickles, and onion and served it to me, dripping down a cardboard takeaway box. I quickly did my Instagram thing and took a bite of what has to be the best quality beef product I've had in a burger.

The fact that all the meat was sourced, butchered, and cooked in-house meant that it was bursting with flavor and juiciness, like nothing I'd ever had before. It didn't take long for me to start telling everyone about it, excitedly, with a hint of obsession.

Eventually, I decided I wanted to do a long-form video with a videographer, showcasing the burger and talking about what made it special. It was then that Chris informed me they'd be adding it to the menu, calling it the "Food Coma Burger." It quickly became a part of my brand and who I am.

Admittedly, I haven't been back to Tender Gourmet Butchery for a little while. Between COVID, the passing of my wife's mother, and my congested work schedule, it has been difficult to drop in. But believe me when I say it—this joint has a special place in the Food Coma genes.

THE 2X2
WINGMILL, NEUTRAL BAY

While there's a crazy world of weird, wacky, and sometimes just downright strange burgers in Sydney, there's also some places that get the fundamentals right, and WingMill is one of them.

My first experience at this place is a bit comical. A week before, I'd had this horrific snowboarding accident that left me with a broken rib and a shattered collarbone. For obvious reasons, I wasn't allowed to drive for two weeks and was relying heavily on the kindness of others. My amazing younger cousin—and recent hire—Samantha, was nice enough to drive me to work that day and look after my fragile ass.

When I rocked up to WingMill, I was in a full sling and had what would have looked like a carer with me (Samantha). Not exactly what they would have been expecting from the Food Coma guy on Instagram.

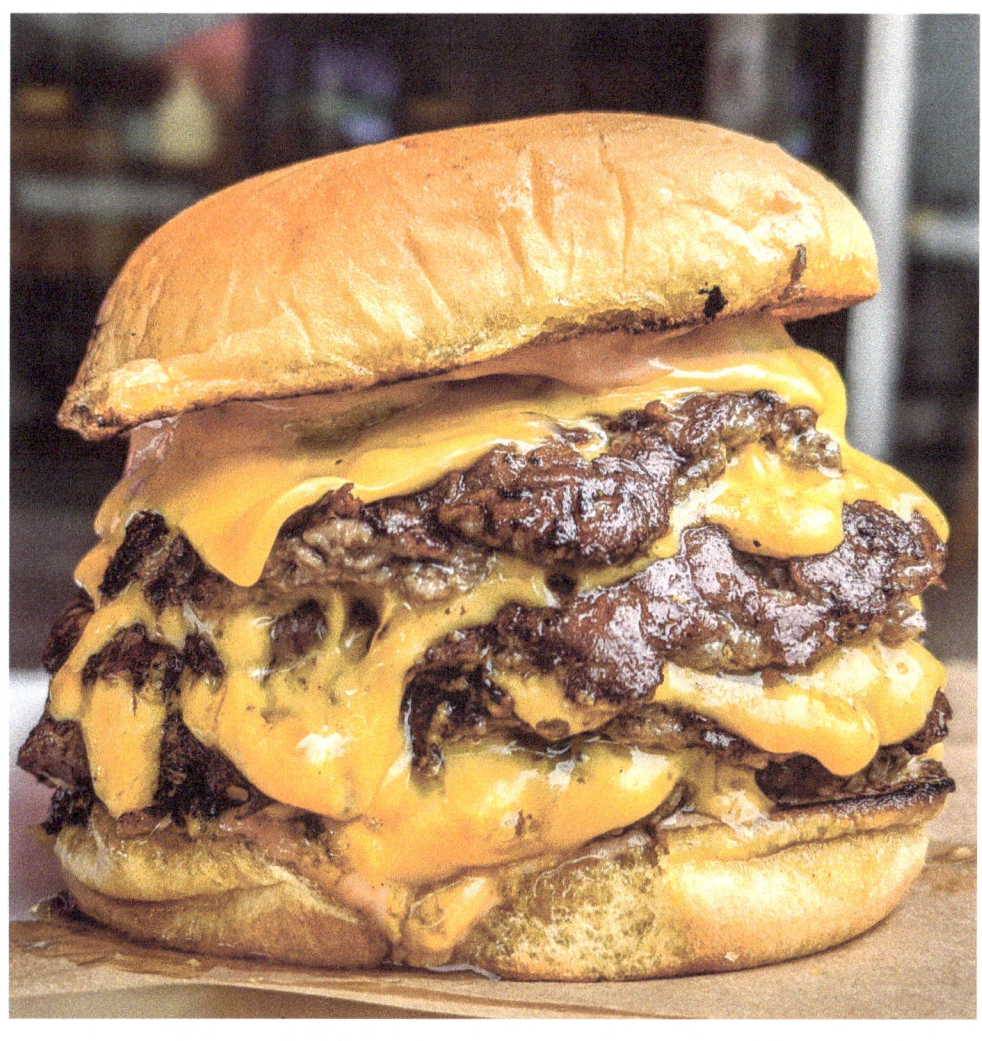

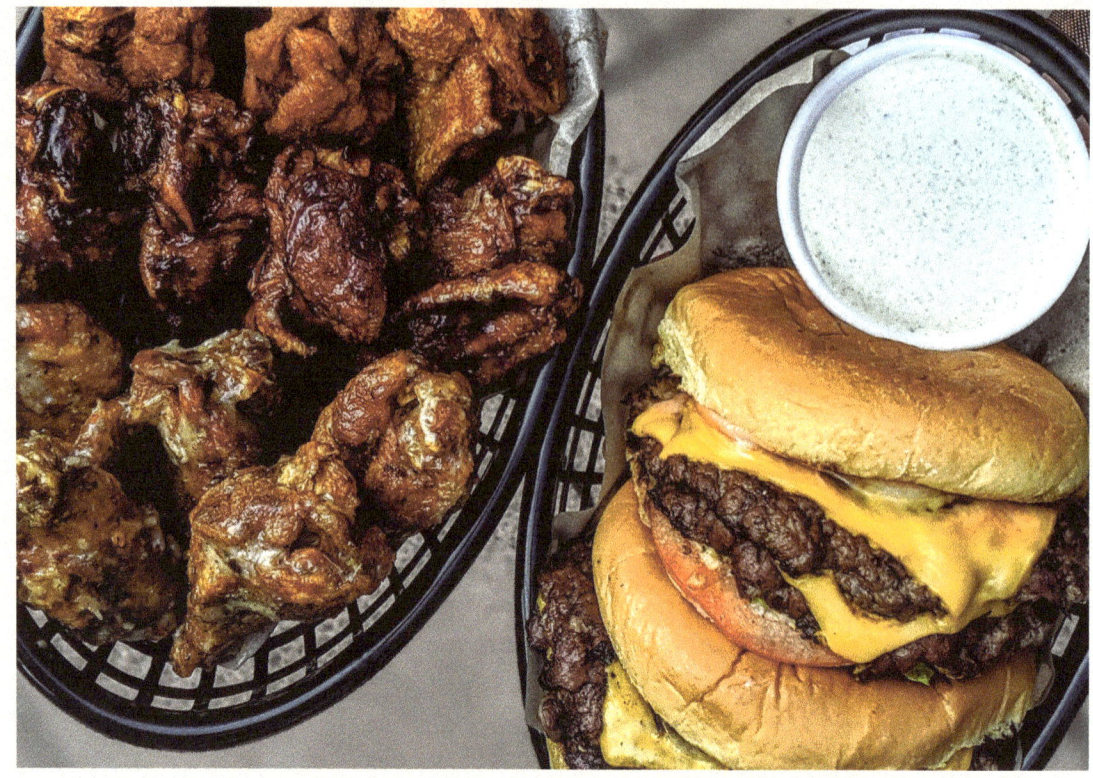

I met Ahmed, the owner of WingMill, and I became hypnotized by his passion. He spoke with electrifying words about his experiences with food, coming from such a humble place of service to others. He had quit his successful career as a car salesman, sold his beautiful Audi, and pursued a career in hospitality—a true sacrifice for a genuine petrol head. We ordered a small assortment of items, and I noticed there was only *one* burger on the menu. I was appalled. It was a bit off-brand for me at the time to not have a crazy, over-the-top burger. But that all changed after this.

The wings came out first, which I still rate as the best I've ever had. Garlic Parmesan wings from WingMill—try them, or you're absolutely lost in life. But then the burger arrived, and it became my favorite simple cheeseburger ever. It was small—again, very off-brand for me at the time—but layered perfectly. It was a delicate and delicious experience that can't be explained without trying it, but I'll do my best.

First, a petite and plushy Martin's Potato Roll, the perfect vessel for a classic combination of sauce, pickles, burger, and vegetables. Thinly sliced shredded iceberg, with just the perfect amount of crunch and freshness without drowning the burger in watery flavors. Two thin slices of tomato, giving a slight pungent and acidic kick. Then a couple of exquisite patties, thinly smashed, seasoned slightly, with a mild mustard grilled in and a warm melted cheese lying tightly on top. Finished with a party of playful pickles on top, with just the right amount of a delicious, pink sauce. If anyone in Sydney asks me for the best place to be introduced to burgers, I always point them in the direction of WingMill.

ALBERTS BURGERS
NORTH SYDNEY (CLOSED)

Once upon a time, a young Jesse attended a university in North Sydney. I was the perfect image of a university student. I surfed in the mornings with my best mate, Simo; I worked 4-5 jobs at a given time, and I attended the gym at ridiculous times of the day, sometimes around midnight. I worked in bars, cafes, delivered food for my local Chinese takeaway, was a surfing and swim coach—the full deal. So, why not add waiter to that list?

At the end of a surfing session with Simo, he mentioned that the pub he worked at was looking for waiters during their hugely busy lunch service. It seemed like a no-brainer for me. Most of my classes finished at lunch and resumed in the afternoon. I'd get a bit of extra cash in hand when I'd usually be wasting time waiting for my next class, and, best of all, I'd get fed at the end of each shift. Ding, ding, ding, we have a winner! The pub was called Alberts, and they had a talented chef there by the name of Andrew. Andrew was a larger-than-life personality, a riot to have a conversation with, and a genuinely nice guy. I didn't know it at the time, but he was quite well-known for making a pretty mean burger.

When I was working, I went about my business, dealing with disgruntled office workers who were fighting it out for a $10 steak or schnitzel, running between the kitchen and tables with food or dirty plates, and attempting to translate the broken English of a couple of the other chefs. The services were hard and fast, a flurry of two hours' worth of chefs shouting, clearing tables, and pouring schooners. Everything would then clear in a matter of minutes, leaving behind a lifeless pub.

When it all ended, Andrew would look over to me with a cheesy grin and ask, "What are you feeling today, mate?"

On one occasion, my best mate floated over and mentioned to me sternly, "You have to try his burgers, best you'll ever have." Well, I trusted him wholeheartedly, so I perused the menu and found a Mexican themed burger. Hell yeah, I could get around that. I ordered it, and it came out in a few minutes. I sat down, took a bite, and all the craziness of the lunch service just melted away. It was my first ever experience of what a proper burger should taste like. I had been exposed to the likes of McDonalds, Hungry Jacks, and a few corner takeaway stores to boot, but nothing like this. It blew me away, and I knew I had found a guilty addiction that would never again be fully itched.

Andrew supported me and my Instagram career for many years after, giving me free food and even hosting an eating competition for me. He eventually opened up in a different hotel and was slinging burgers for quite a while. Sadly, he has since hung up the apron and moved on to other things, but I am lucky enough to be one of the many who were able to experience his burgers.

THE FORGETABOUDIT
CRINITI'S

I write this with a word of warning: in no way was this the best burger I'd ever had, nor was it even in the top 200. But Criniti's was a part of the beginning of everything for me, and I was lucky enough to have been able to make the most of my time there.

Many years ago, I had just started my competitive eating journey. The first victim to fall to my iron gut was 1 kg of veal schnitzel and four sides from Bavarian Bier Cafe. But my second victim was the one that started everything for me: the 1-meter pizza challenge at Criniti's.

I was living in North Manly at the time, halfway through my degree, doing my best to make ends meet. After cruising through my first ever food challenge, I knew I could set the bar higher, and another food challenge across the road caught my eye. One meter of pizza, one hour, with the grand prize being FREE FOOD FOR A YEAR! Those words sang like angels in my ears. It was an opportunity for me to save some money and have fun in the process. I started to spread the word among family and friends.

I began my first ever competitive eating training, eating huge bowls of cooked vegetables, then drinking water until my stomach felt like it was going to burst. I'd go through whole packets of gum, chewing and gnawing until my jaw felt like it was hanging down by my ankles. I'd exercise constantly, building up my appetite and fitness, trying to gain every bit of competitive advantage. Finally, I set a date and invited my family and friends along to witness this strange activity called "competitive eating."

I sat there, nervous, fighting off tiredness (I had been fasting for about twenty-four hours), scrolling through Instagram, looking at food to hype myself up. Finally, the pizza came out of the oven, steam cascading across it as it arrived at my table. An animal awoke within me, and I couldn't hold back any longer. I attacked the pizza, showing no regard for any of the other guests at the restaurant. The first slice hit my mouth, and hot, molten cheese stuck immediately to the roof of my mouth. I had tunnel vision and barely noticed, continuing to gnaw, bite, and slurp my way through kilograms of pizza. It wasn't long before I started to notice the pain growing in the roof of my mouth, each slice of pizza scratching along my burned gums, like sandpaper on a piece of soft fruit. I kept my cool and soldiered on with my eyes on the prize. After twenty-two minutes, I gingerly finished the last mouthful, absolutely spent. I got a round of applause and slowly walked, hunched over, to the table of friends and family, trying not to aggravate my stomach.

After half an hour of holding back kilograms of pizza, I needed to leave and get fresh air. I walked at snail's pace to the pedestrian crossing, where I immediately halted. Shallow breaths were the only thing keeping my pizza inside me as I waited for the feeling to subside. I was finally able to cross and walk my way over to the nearby park. I sat there in a daze for an hour as my friends sat chatting excitedly about what they had just witnessed. It was finally over.

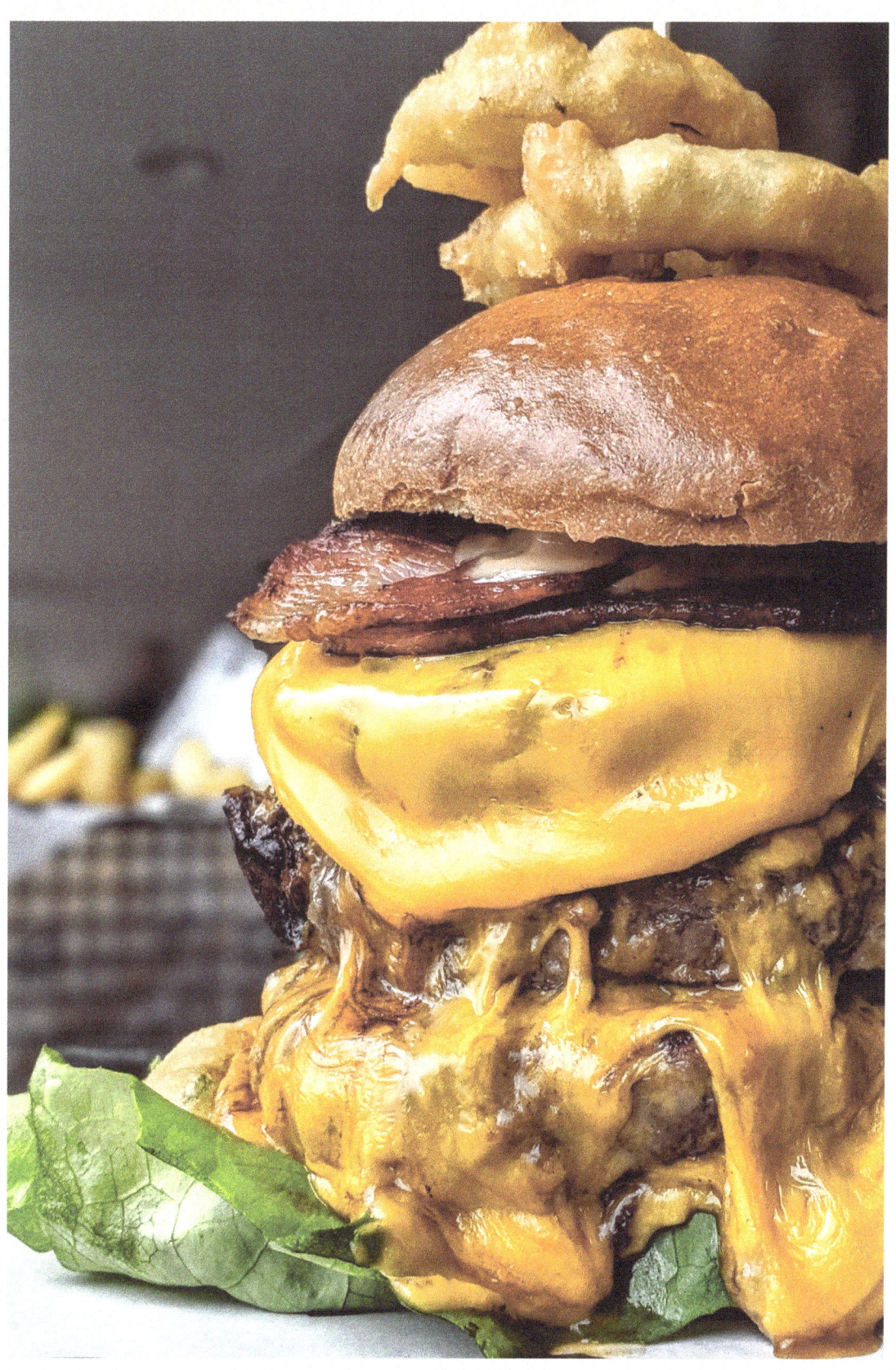

I had held the food in and completed the challenge.

It was time to collect my prize: a year's worth of food. The terms and conditions stated that it was to be one dining experience per week, with an entree, main, and dessert comped, as long as I had a guest that purchased a main meal, which we would split. This seemed quite reasonable to me, and I started to view it as an opportunity. Is there not a more intimate experience than having a one-on-one dinner with a friend or family member? I didn't think so. So, I devised a plan to invite a new friend or family member every week to have dinner with me. I had no idea what this experience would awaken within me.

It was the most wonderful opportunity I'd had in my entire life. I wasn't particularly wealthy, sometimes just scraping by week to week, and, as a result, it was hard to be generous to people with anything but my time and favors. But now I was able to give back to the people who had been such a deep part of my life and have rare conversations that are only achievable during such an intimate experience. I'd take a new person each week, and we would talk about our aspirations, work quarrels, difficulties, and hobbies. They were deep conversations, always respectful and loving, that covered a range of topics. It made me realize what a powerful tool quality time is, regardless of whether it's in a restaurant or not.

Gradually, I got to know the staff, managers, and waiters, learning about their lives, where they'd come from, where they'd been, and where they planned to go. Eventually, I knew them all by name and learned just how amazing each individual was.

It also kickstarted my love for food photography. Each time, I'd whip out my phone and take pictures of the food we ate and the people I was with. Eventually, Criniti's was where I took my parents (together) and convinced them I could make a run at this Instagram world.

Oh yeah, during those dinners, I'd order a burger called the Forgetaboudit because it was the biggest burger they had, and it filled me up. That's all I really have to say about that.

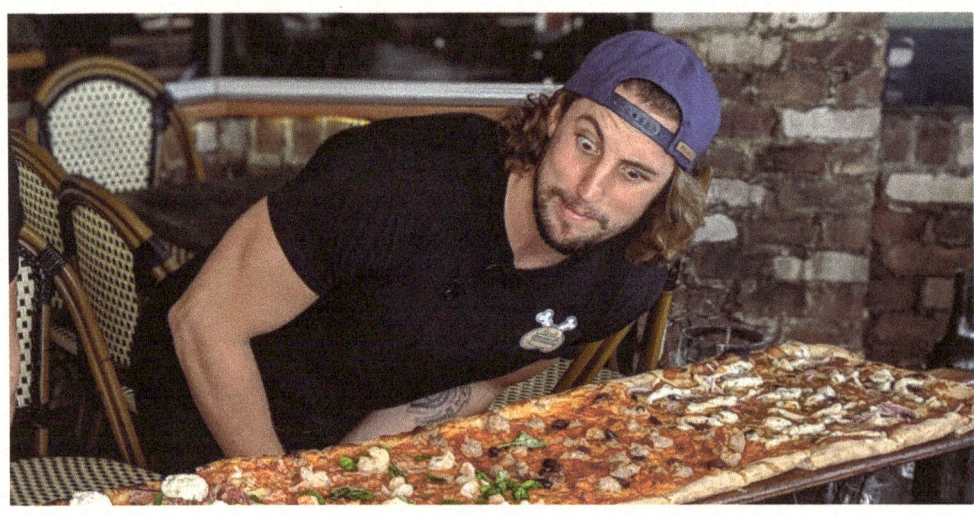

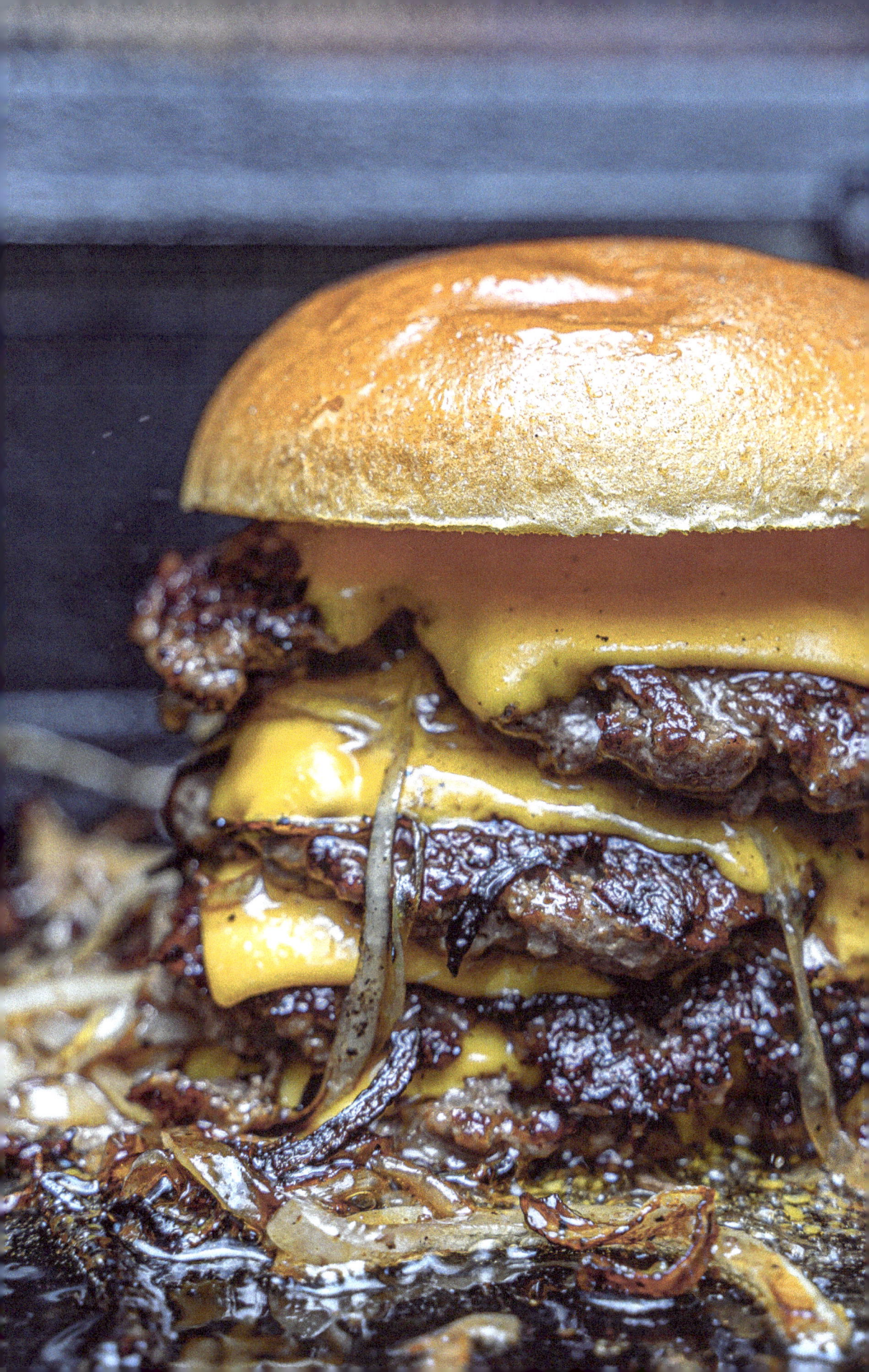

ACKNOWLEDGMENTS

I'd like to start by giving HUGE props to the entire hospitality industry after COVID-19. You guys are rockstars, on the frontline every day, feeding people despite the danger it brought you. You persisted through what was undeniably one of the most heartbreaking moments in your careers.

To all the chefs, for giving me the time of day, humoring my questions and sharing in my excitement. You guys inspired me to be better every day. You are gladiators of the hospitality world. You go to war with a service from the time you start prepping, all the way till you're scrubbing and cleaning at the end of a hard night.

To one of my best mates, Loch. Thank you for being the catalyst for my competitive eating career. You inspired me and helped me start something huge. I enjoyed every day we did it together.

To all of my friends, thank you for your patience with me. Attempting this journey has meant I have been absent numerous times, which has been difficult. You guys give me the energy and passion I need every day. I see you like family, and I am glad I can give back more time now.

To my lovely parents, Kerrie and Mark. Thank you for believing in me. You didn't push me toward a traditional career, but instead trusted in my judgment. Our long conversations about business and growth have always challenged me and enabled me to grow. You brought me up in such a way that helped me maintain integrity and passion throughout every career I've undertaken. You are amazing.

To my Wife, Kira. You have been a trooper for the duration of our relationship. I was absent with long work hours and my face buried in my laptop or phone around you. The loss of your mother could have broken you, but instead I've seen an independent and beautiful person emerge. I hope I can continue to repay the favor until we are old and wrinkly.

To my in-laws, Anna and Paul. Paul, thank you for letting me marry your daughter. You never questioned my ability to provide and always trusted me to love her. You've helped me grow as a husband and shown me what a great dad you can be. Anna, bloody hell I miss you. You were such a rock for so many people. I miss talking about food with you and sharing recipes.

You were always so interested in everything I was doing, and you were one of the most generous people I know.

I believe it's nearly impossible to get an acknowledgment right. Because every person in your journey has some sort of impact on you. Every person I've spoken to has given me inspiration. So, it's almost bittersweet putting one together. I wish I could mention every person for every little thing, but that'd be a book on its own. So, let's settle for this for now then, shall we?

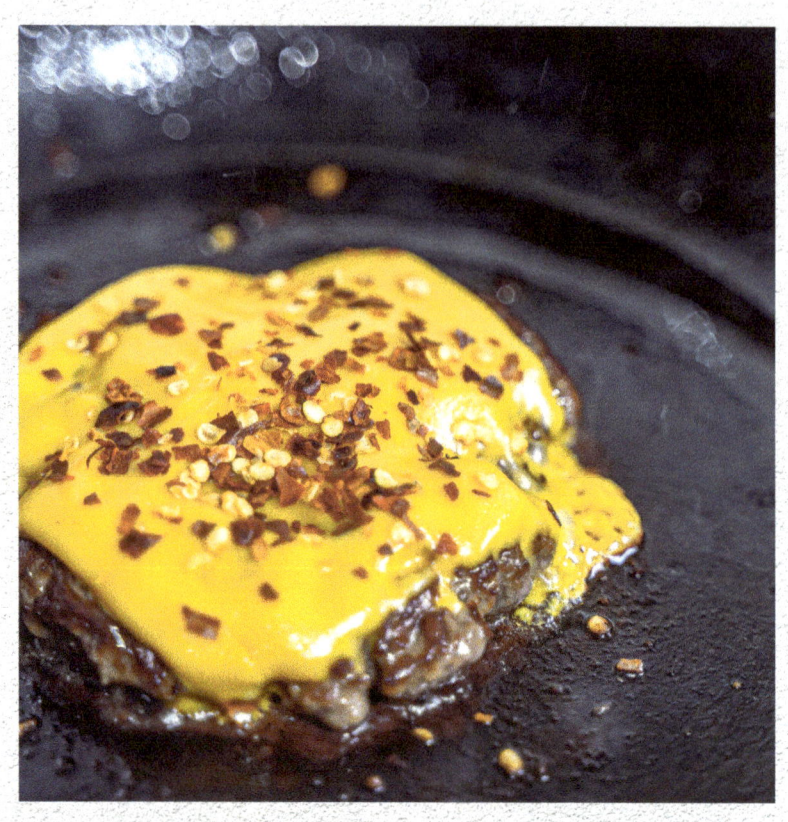

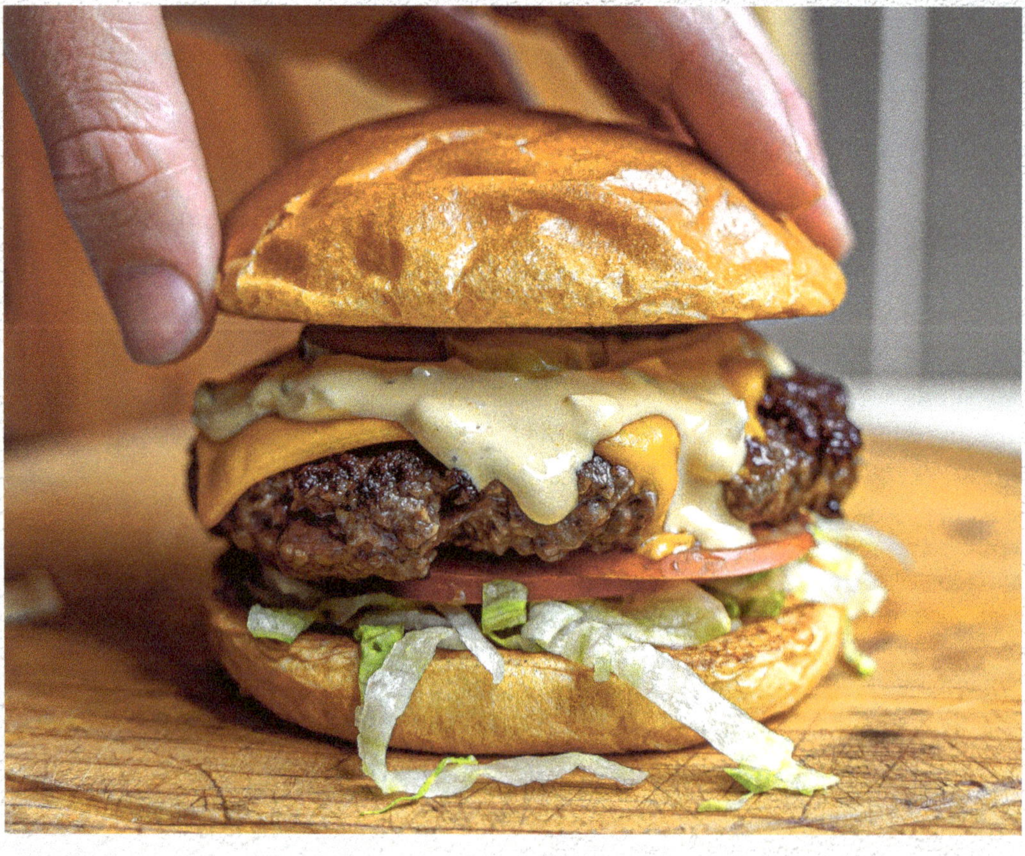

ABOUT THE AUTHOR

Jesse Freeman, the creator of @foodcoma_eats on Instagram, has been headfirst in the hospitality industry since a young age: from starting his journey as a barista and bartender in his formative years, to his commitment to a Sydney-based food blog, to finally the documenting of his home cooking journey. Jesse used his many years working for and with hospitality businesses to cultivate his cooking knowledge, better understand the basics, and experiment from there.

Beginning his blogging career as a YouTube-based competitive eater, Jesse walked away with a cult following for his crazy antics and big eating feats. Reaching his peak as a two-time Guinness world record holder for eating, after traveling across Australia competing, Jesse then focused his efforts on the growth of his Instagram and his work within the hospitality industry. He traveled across NSW, visiting businesses, helping them grow their social profile and learning about everything hospitality, including suppliers, operations, staffing, and cooking techniques. After many years sharing his obsession of hospitality with the world, he started his home cooking journey on Instagram. From here, he built a strong following of people interested in the intricacies of cooking burgers and then progressed to other savory cuisines.

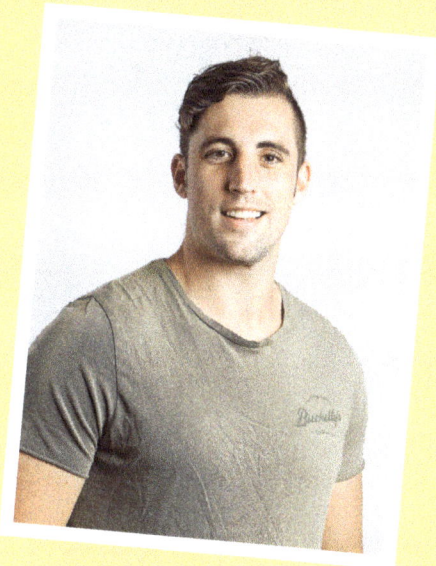

After a couple of largely successful pop-ups, he has shown the world that he's got the passion and know-how to serve people his food.

**ARE YOU READY TO JOIN ME
ON MY BURGER JOURNEY?**

**ADD ME ON SOCIALS TO BECOME
A PART OF THE FOOD COMA FAMILY.**

EPIC VIDEOS, EXCLUSIVE CONTENT, OUTRAGEOUS
CREATIONS—AND IT'S NOT JUST BURGERS EITHER.
I'M TALKING HOME COOKING TAKEN TO THE EXTREME
AND PLENTY OF LOCAL FEEDS FOR ADDED FLAVOR.

IF YOU'RE A FAN OF GREAT FOOD—WHO ISN'T?—
I'D LOVE TO HAVE YOU ALONG FOR THE RIDE.

LET'S DO THIS!

**PERSONAL INSTAGRAM: @JESSEFREEMAN
BUSINESS: @FOODCOMA_EATS
YOUTUBE: YOUTUBE.COM/FOODCOMA**

www.ingramcontent.com/pod-product-compliance
Lightning Source LLC
Chambersburg PA
CBHW041219240426
43661CB00012B/1088